HOW PSYCHOTHERAPY WORKS

HOW PSYCHOTHERAPY WORKS
Process and Technique

Joseph Weiss

FOREWORD BY
Harold Sampson, Ph.D.

GUILFORD PRESS

New York   London

Library of Congress Cataloging-in-Publication Data

Weiss, Joseph
    How psychotherapy works : process and technique / Joseph Weiss ;
foreword by Harold Sampson.
        p. cm.
    Includes bibliographical references and index.
    ISBN 0–89862–548–3
    1. Psychotherapy. I. Title.
    [DNLM: 1. Psychotherapy—methods. 2. Psychoanalytic Theory. WM
420 W4312h 1993]
    RC480.5.W355 1993
    616.89'14—dc20
    DNLM/DLC
    for Library of Congress   93-25473
                                                                              CIP

Foreword

In an exciting and highly original work, Weiss presents an elegant and powerful theory of therapy that has been tested by both clinical observation and research studies. The theory casts new light on how psychotherapy works. The principles of technique that follow from the theory are illustrated with carefully selected and diverse clinical examples.

Weiss assumes that persons are powerfully motivated, from infancy onward, to understand their reality and to adapt to it. In working to do so, they develop, by inference from experience, beliefs about their reality—including, most importantly, beliefs about themselves and their interpersonal world. Some of these beliefs are "pathogenic" in that they impede functioning, adversely affect self-esteem, and prevent the person from pursuing normal, desirable goals. Pathogenic beliefs warn the person who holds them that the pursuit of desirable goals—for example, to be independent, happy, or relaxed, or to have a good marriage or satisfying career—will endanger the person or others. To avoid these dangers, the person may renounce valued goals, and may develop inhibitions and symptoms. Psychopathology stems from pathogenic beliefs.

Weiss's theory of therapy follows directly from this account of the patient's problems. Psychotherapy is a process in which the patient works to disconfirm his pathogenic beliefs with the help of the therapist. The person is powerfully motivated to disconfirm these beliefs because they are grim and maladaptive, cause the person to sacrifice desired goals, and produce much suffering. Patients work throughout therapy to disprove these beliefs and to overcome the problems to which they give rise. Patients work by unconsciously testing their pathogenic beliefs in relation to the therapist. They also work to become conscious (with the help of interpretations) of their pathogenic beliefs, and to recognize that these beliefs are irrational and maladaptive. A patient's work is guided by unconscious goals and plans, and his progress is regulated by unconscious appraisals of danger and safety. Patients lift repressions and make therapeutic progress when they believe they may do so safely.

The task of the therapist is to help the patient in his struggle to disprove pathogenic beliefs and to pursue the goals forbidden by them. The therapist may do this in many ways. He may help the patient to disconfirm pathogenic beliefs by his overall attitude toward the patient; he may do so by passing the patient's tests; he may do so by interpretations. The therapist must adapt his approach to each patient's particular pathogenic beliefs and goals.

This outline cannot do justice to the theory, nor to the richness and subtlety of its clinical applications. This said, I would nonetheless emphasize that because of the theory's clarity and coherence, its fundamental propositions can be set forth intelligibly, even in outline form. Weiss's theory has the simplicity that is desirable for any good theory: Its basic propositions are internally consistent, and give order to a wide range of phenomena within its domain.

Weiss developed this theory through studies of process notes of psychoanalyses, and later of psychotherapies. He sought to find out what actually brings about significant therapeutic changes—such as the patient's becoming aware of previously repressed ideas or memories, manifesting new affects, developing new insights into his conscious and unconscious life, or displaying new capacities in his behavior. His empirical approach led to the observation that analytic patients were often calm when previously repressed material emerged, and they did not seem to be in conflict with this material. Many familiar psychoanalytic hypotheses could not account well for these and other related observations. Weiss gradually developed new hypotheses that provided a better fit to the observations and appeared to have considerable explanatory power. Many of these hypotheses have been tested and supported by rigorous research studies carried out over the past 20 or more years.

The theory derives its clinical power not only from its empirical origin and closeness to observation, but also from Weiss's cogent exposition of how to infer, from the patient's history and behavior in treatment, what the patient is trying to accomplish, and how the therapist may help the patient to do this. In addition, the theory enables the therapist to identify accurately lawful relations in the unfolding therapeutic process, and to observe previously unnoticed connections between the therapist's attitude and behavior and subsequent patient material.

For example, a female patient unconsciously believed that the therapist would want to criticize her accomplishments as her father had done. She tested this belief in an early session by saying that although she had laid out her problems fairly well, she was being too intellectual and was probably avoiding something. The therapist questioned the patient's self-criticism of her performance during the session. She did not reply directly but somewhat later in the session she spontaneously recalled a childhood incident. Her father had pointed out to her that a school paper about which she had felt pride had not addressed certain issues and was therefore inadequate. The patient began the next session by talking for the first time about how good she was at her research work. Weiss's concepts enabled this therapist to see the connection between the patient's claim that she was avoiding something, his questioning of her claim, her subsequent spontaneous recall of a childhood memory of her father criticizing her accomplishments, and the patient's talking of her work achievements in the next session. The patient tested her pathogenic belief first by inviting the therapist to agree with her self-criticism. When he did not do so, she began to recall something of the origins of the particular belief. In the next hour, she tested the therapist by describing her accomplishments with pride, inviting the therapist to challenge her (and hoping he would not).

This vignette, like many examples in the book, illustrates how Weiss's theory orients the therapist about what is happening, and how it enables him to test out his understanding of the patient and the treatment process. In the preceding example, the therapist could observe the helpfulness of his intervention. In other instances, the therapist may observe that his intervention is not helpful, as shown by subsequent patient material. The therapist can then correct his understanding of the patient and the therapy, and adapt his interventions to better fit the patient's needs.

Weiss challenges many familiar ideas about psychotherapy—for example, such ideas as that the patient's primary motivation in therapy is to avoid facing his problems or to gratify infantile wishes; or that the patient's reenactments in therapy are primarily attempts at gratification or defense; or that the therapist's neutrality is essential to fundamental change; or that the patient's dreams are primary-process expressions of repressed wishes; or that the corrective emotional experience prevents fundamental changes from taking place. In some instances, Weiss fits a familiar idea into broader principles of technique. This enables Weiss to show how and when the idea is useful, and how and when it may be misleading. For example, Weiss shows that analytic neutrality is useful when it disconfirms the patient's pathogenic beliefs, but that in other instances it may tend to support certain pathogenic beliefs, and interfere with the patient's progress.

Weiss's approach transcends a number of familiar dichotomies (and, correspondingly, familiar controversies) by focusing on more fundamental processes. For example, Weiss has demonstrated that any intervention that disconfirms a pathogenic belief—whether it be supportive or interactive or interpretive—will reduce the patient's sense of danger and therefore lessen his need for repression. Interventions such as encouragement or reassurance enable certain patients to lift their repressions, to develop new insights into their unconscious mental lives, and to relinquish inhibitions and symptoms. As Weiss points out, such observations deprive the dichotomy of "supportive versus uncovering" therapies of much of its significance. Weiss's point applies equally to such dichotomies as "interactive versus interpretive" therapies, or "relational versus analytic" therapies.

Although Weiss's theory challenges many of Freud's early ideas about unconscious mental functioning, psychopathology, and treatment, he shows that his work stems from certain concepts in Freuds later writings. His theory has important links to many other developments in psychoanalytic thought. Weiss has not been directly influenced by Sullivan's interpersonal theory or by such object relations theorists as Fairbairn and Winnicott, but his work shares important thematic congruences with (and also shares important differences from) their contributions. These congruences include the idea that the infant has a primary motivation, independent of drives, to seek and maintain object relationships, that the seeking of pleasure or gratification is subordinate to seeking and maintaining the all important ties to the parents; that psychopathology is based on efforts to adapt to one's reality; that compliances with environmental demands may be an important source of psychopathology, and that children may deny or distort reality for the adaptive purpose of protecting their relationship to their parents. Weiss's theory is also compatible with aspects of Bowlby's attachment theory, with findings in contemporary psychoanalytic research on infant development, and with other contemporary analytic work.

The theory is also relevant for the nonanalytic theorist or practitioner, because of the theory's emphasis on the centrality of adaptation; on the importance of the patient's sense of safety to therapeutic progress; and on the role of higher mental functions, such as beliefs, in psychopathology and treatment. As an example, nonanalytic as well as analytic theorists and practitioners concerned with the treatment of patients abused in childhood can find much in Weiss's work that is congenial and useful. Moreover, this is a two-way street: Weiss's theory has the structure, through its concepts of pathology stemming from pathogenic beliefs and treatment consisting of the disconfirmation of those beliefs, to incorporate readily the valuable ideas and discoveries of specialists in these areas.

I believe that this book is a major contribution that will transform the reader's thinking about, and doing, psychotherapy. It will also change the reader's ideas and intuitions about human nature, basic motivations, the unconscious mind, and psychopathology. I trust that it will have a similar impact on the development of our field.

HAROLD SAMPSON

Preface and
Acknowledgments

A few years ago, Harold Sampson, myself, and Mount Zion Psychotherapy Research Group (now known as the San Francisco Psychotherapy Research Group) presented a distinctive psychoanalytic theory of the mind, psychopathology, and therapy, for which we found support through numerous formal quantitative research studies (Weiss, Sampson, and the Mount Zion Psychotherapy Research Group, 1986). The theory is distinctive in its emphasis on concepts that Freud developed in his late works concerning the patient's unconscious cognition, his unconscious problem-solving activities, and his powerful unconscious wish to master his problems (see Chapter 9). The theory has broad implications for the understanding of human behavior, and it bears on the techniques of psychoanalysis and psychoanalytic psychotherapy.

In this book, in which I develop the implications of my theory for technique, I have included numerous clinical examples. These are intended to illustrate my concepts, not to provide convincing evidence for them. I have presented my examples simply and directly in the hope that by making my meanings explicit, I will enable readers to think about my concepts and decide whether or not to agree with them. I have derived my ideas from research and clinical observation and invite readers to do their own research on them, informally by clinical observation or by use of formal research methods.

Because of our conviction about the importance of research, Harold Sampson and I founded the Mount Zion Psychotherapy Research Group in 1972 in order to test the validity of my concepts by formal quantitative research methods. Since then, as co-directors of this group, we have supervised numerous such studies of these concepts. The ideas that the patient's psychopathology stems from unconscious pathogenic beliefs; that the patient is highly motivated to disprove these beliefs; and that he works in therapy according to simple plans to accomplish this. We have also demonstrated that the patient exerts considerable control over his unconscious mental life. Our research has helped me and my collaborators to develop and refine the theory.

In Chapter 8 of this book I present a number of our research studies. This chapter contains studies not included in *The Psychoanalytic Process* (Weiss et al., 1986), and it is written for the clinician who does not have special knowledge of research methods.

In developing my concepts of the mind, theory, and technique, I am extremely indebted to Harold Sampson. We have been collaborating since 1964, and have discussed theory, therapy, and technique regularly since then. Hal's lucid thinking and his broad and detailed perspective on psychology and psychoanalysis have been of inestimable help to me.

Our research has been greatly enriched by the work of John Curtis and George Silberschatz, who collected and transcribed a large number of brief, time-limited (16-session) psychotherapies. Curtis and Silberschatz have not only studied these psychotherapies themselves; they have supervised the study of these therapies by a number of investigators, who under their guidance have carried out significant investigations.

Tom Kelly and Jack Berry have helped us a great deal in the statistical analysis of our research data. I am indebted to both of them. I am also greatly indebted to Lynn O'Connor, who from the beginning has discussed with me the organization of the book. She has brought to my attention the kind of material that the psychology student may find useful. Moreover, my thinking has been enriched by our clinical and theoretical discussions.

Jessica Broitman, Marshall Bush, Ted Dorpat, Steve Frankel, Suzanne Gassner, Kathy Mulherin, and Denny Zeitlin have read my entire manuscript and made many useful suggestions. Estelle Weiss has carefully edited the entire manuscript, line by line, thereby making it more readable. My editor at The Guilford Press, Kitty Moore, has helped me in the organization of the book and encouraged me to include certain topics that I had omitted. Michael Simon has carried out many tasks essential to the production of this book. And finally, Kelly McMullen and Erin Merritt have cheerfully and competently typed and retyped the manuscript.

Contents

PART 1

THE TECHNIQUE OF PSYCHOTHERAPY: THEORY AND PRACTICE

CHAPTER 1

Introduction

The subject of this book is the technique of psychotherapy. The concepts about technique presented here are based on a psychoanalytic theory that contains distinctive ideas about unconscious mental functioning, motivation, and psychopathology.

This theory assumes that the patient's problems stem from frightening unconscious maladaptive beliefs, here called "pathogenic," that impede his[1] functioning, adversely affect his self-esteem, and prevent his pursuit of highly adaptive and desirable goals (e.g., happiness, success, or a good relationship). The patient suffers from these beliefs and is powerfully motivated both consciously and unconsciously to disprove them, and he works with the therapist to do this. The therapist's basic task follows from these assumptions: It is to help the patient in his efforts to disprove the beliefs and to pursue the goals they warn him against.

The theory outlined above is Freudian in that it is based on certain ideas about the mind, motivation, psychopathology, and therapy that Freud developed in a piecemeal and unsystematic fashion as parts of his ego psychology (see Chapter 9 for a discussion of this development). However, as I discuss later, it is based on quite different theoretical assumptions from those presented by Freud in his *Papers on Technique* (1911–1915).

[1]For the sake of brevity and readability, the masculine pronoun is used in its generic sense throughout this book.

The technical ideas proposed here are broad enough to apply both to psychoanalysis and to psychoanalytic psychotherapy. This account deals with what these therapies have in common; how they differ is beyond the scope of this book. In this and the next chapter, I prepare the reader for my technical ideas by reviewing the theory on which they are based.

A REVIEW OF BASIC THEORY

Motivation

A person's most powerful motivation is to adapt to reality, especially the reality of his interpersonal world. He begins in infancy and early childhood to work at adapting to his interpersonal world, and he continues to do this throughout life. As part of this effort, he seeks reliable beliefs (knowledge) about himself and his world. He works throughout life to learn how he affects others and how others are likely to react to him. He also works to learn the moral and ethical assumptions that others will expect him to abide by in his relations with them, and that they will abide by in their relations with him. He begins in infancy to learn about these things both by inference from experience with his parents and siblings, and by their teachings.

A person's beliefs about reality and morality are central to his conscious and unconscious mental life. These beliefs are endowed with awesome authority. They guide the all-important tasks of adaptation and self-preservation. They organize perception; a person perceives himself and others largely as he believes himself and others to be. In addition, such beliefs organize personality. It is in accordance with his beliefs about reality and morality that a person shapes his strivings, affects, and moods, and by doing so evolves his personality. Moreover, it is in obedience to certain maladaptive beliefs, here called "pathogenic," that a person develops and maintains his psychopathology.

Unconscious Mental Functioning

A person may carry out unconsciously many of the same kinds of functions that he carries out consciously. He may think,

make inferences, test reality, and make and carry out decisions and plans. Moreover, he may exert some control over his unconscious mental life in accordance with these decisions and plans. In regulating his unconscious mental life, he is especially concerned with seeking safety and avoiding danger. He regulates his repressions and his inhibitions in accordance with this concern. He maintains the repression of a mental content as long as he unconsciously assumes that experiencing it would endanger him. He lifts the repression of the content when he decides he may safely experience it.

The idea that a person represses, or suppresses, certain unconscious mental contents until he unconsciously judges that he may safely experience them may be illustrated by the phenomenon of crying at the happy ending (Weiss, 1952, 1971; Weiss, Sampson, & the Mount Zion Psychotherapy Research Group, 1986). A good instance of this is provided by the moviegoer who suppresses his sadness while the lovers in the movie quarrel, but weeps when they reconcile. The moviegoer suppresses his sadness while the lovers are quarreling, because he feels endangered by it. However, at the movie's happy ending, when he no longer has reason to feel sad, he permits himself to experience the sadness.

The moviegoer's sadness is not deeply repressed. However, in everyday life a person in a happy ending may bring forth deeply repressed sadness connected with painful traumatic events. For example, Roberta P. (a patient whom I discuss in Chapter 3) after feeling accepted by the therapist became happy and at the same time brought forth deeply repressed sad memories of maternal rejection.

Psychopathology

Psychopathology is rooted in pathogenic beliefs; these are compelling, grim, and maladaptive. They warn the person guided by them that if he attempts to pursue certain normal, desirable goals, such as a satisfying career or a happy marriage, he will endanger himself or others. He fears external dangers such as the disruption of an important relationship, or internal dangers such as a painful affect (e.g., fear, anxiety, guilt, shame, or remorse). It is in obedience to his pathogenic beliefs and the dangers they warn him against that a person maintains his repressions and inhibitions. He represses the goals he believes to be dangerous, and he inhibits himself from pursuing these goals.

A person develops pathogenic beliefs in childhood by inferring them from traumatic experiences with parents and siblings. These are experiences in which he finds that by attempting to attain a normal, desirable goal, he brings about a disruption in his ties to his parents. For example, he may infer that he burdens his parents by being dependent on them, or that he causes them to feel hurt and rejected by being independent of them.

The Power of Pathogenic Beliefs

The power of pathogenic beliefs derives from the fact that they are acquired in infancy and early childhood from parents and siblings, whom the child endows with absolute authority. His parents are critically important to him because he needs them in order to survive and flourish. His only good strategy for adaptation is to develop and maintain a reliable relationship with them. Because his parents are so important to him, he is highly motivated to perceive them as all-powerful and wise. Moreover, he has no prior knowledge of human relations by which to judge them. Therefore, when in conflict with his parents, he tends to perceive them as right and himself as wrong. This has been demonstrated by Beres (1958) in a research study of children placed in foster homes. In each instance, the child assumed that he had been sent away as a punishment for something bad he had done, and that the punishment was deserved.

Just how a child who is placed away from home blames himself for parental rejection depends on several factors, including how in his opinion he upset his parents before they rejected him. For example, a child whose parents were persistently angered by his demands may infer that he was rejected for being too demanding. Or a child whose parents blamed him for his assertiveness may infer that he was rejected for being too assertive.

Since pathogenic beliefs develop in early childhood, they are concerned with the motivations of the young child in relation to his parents. These include the child's wishes to depend on his parents, to trust them, to be able to be independent of them, to compete with them, and to identify with them. The child may infer and so come to believe that almost any important impulse, attitude, or goal, if experienced or acted upon, will put him in a situation of danger.

The dangers that the child's beliefs warn him against may be internal or external. He may assume that if he pursues a forbidden goal he will suffer fear, shame, remorse, or self-torment, or that he will bring about a serious disruption in his relations with his parents. He may expect to hurt them or to be rejected or punished by them.

Pathogenic beliefs reflect the child's egocentricity, his lack of knowledge of causality, and his ignorance of human relations. The child tends to take responsibility for whatever he experiences. He may take responsibility for anything unfavorable that a parent does, or for anything unfortunate that happens to a parent. For example, he may take responsibility for the depression, illness, or death of a parent, or for the unfavorable ways his parents treat each other.

One boy of $2\frac{1}{2}$ was sent away for 5 months to live with an uncle and aunt, because his parents were overwhelmed by the task of taking care of his sick younger brother and were afraid that the boy would catch the disease. However, the boy believed that he was sent away because his restless activity had burdened his mother. He complied with this belief by becoming especially docile and passive, and he remained this way long after he came back to live with his parents. As a consequence of his mother's sending him away, this boy acquired a number of other pathogenic beliefs: He inferred that his mother was ruthless and powerful; that if he defied her she would mete out swift, hostile punishment; and that she was untrustworthy. Finally, he acquired the pathogenic belief that if he were complacent, relaxed, and happy, something catastrophic would befall him.

A child may take much more responsibility for his parents than is justified by his real power to affect them. A young child whose mother is chronically depressed may assume that he has the power to make her happy, and he may try desperately to cheer her up (see Zahn-Waxler & Radke-Yarrow, 1982). A child whose parents are withdrawn and self-centered may assume that if he were only more engaging he would arouse their interest. A child whose parents are neurotically worried about him may assume that their worry is justified by his defects.

Means of Acquiring Pathogenic Beliefs

A child may acquire pathogenic beliefs simply by assuming that the ways his parents treat him are the ways he should be treated. For instance, a patient in childhood had experienced herself as "low man on the totem pole." Her father, a hard-working minister of a large congregation, spent little time with her. Her mother, who was somewhat depressed, had been more interested in the patient's vivacious older sister than in the more docile patient. The patient developed the idea that she deserved to be treated as unimportant. In her analysis, she felt uncomfortable about complaining, making demands, or taking herself seriously. In her marriage, she accepted the little that her husband and children gave her as all she deserved.

A child may also develop pathogenic beliefs by instruction from his parents. Consider, for example, a patient whose mother repeatedly told him that he belonged to her and that he should sacrifice his interests for hers. He consciously repudiated this idea but unconsciously accepted it, and even as an adult he continued to behave in accordance with it. He worked hard for little money or pleasure, and he married a woman who demanded much but gave little (Asch, 1976).

Sometimes a child develops pathogenic beliefs from accidental events. A patient who at age 4 was kept in bed 6 months for treatment of an orthopedic disease acquired the pathogenic belief that he should not enjoy "charging ahead." As an adult he continued to comply with this belief. After periods of happy and successful activity, he would become depressed and relatively inactive. A patient whose mother had died when the patient was 9 developed the pathogenic belief that she did not deserve a good mother–child relationship. In her adult life she complied with this belief by pulling away from her daughters when she found herself enjoying them.

A child may develop pathogenic beliefs from either "strain" traumas or "shock" traumas. A child incurs a strain trauma over a long period of time in a pathogenic relationship with a parent. For example, a boy whose father rarely spoke to him was traumatized by his father's taciturnity; he blamed himself for it and developed the belief that he did not deserve to be spoken to. A child incurs a shock trauma from a sudden overwhelming event, such as placement away from home or the unexpected illness or death of a parent. The child is prone to take responsibility for such an event, and thus to develop pathogenic beliefs from it by retrospective inference. He assumes after the event that he brought it about by attempting to seek certain goals, to maintain certain attitudes, or to exercise certain functions.

THE PATIENT'S UNCONSCIOUS WORK

A person suffers from pathogenic beliefs and is highly motivated to disprove them. Throughout therapy he works with the therapist to do this. He unconsciously tests these beliefs with his therapist, and he uses the therapist's interpretations to become conscious of the beliefs and to realize that they are false and maladaptive. *The therapeutic process is the process by which the patient works with the therapist at the task of disconfirming his pathogenic beliefs.*

The patient works to change his pathogenic beliefs in an orderly way: He makes simple plans (which are in varying degrees unconscious) about which problems to tackle during a particular phase of treatment and which ones to defer tackling until later. In addition, he takes into account the dangers predicted by the beliefs, and the painful affects to which the beliefs give rise. Also, he takes into account his abilities and his current reality, which includes his assessment of the therapist. He may in some instances decide not to tackle his more difficult problems at the beginning, but to work to acquire the strength to tackle them later. If at the beginning he believes himself especially threatened by a particular danger, he may, as illustrated below, begin therapy by working to assure himself that this danger is not real.

Sylvia G.

Sylvia G. came to analysis because she had difficulty feeling close to her husband. This difficulty stemmed from her pathogenic belief that she was responsible for him. She assumed that her husband, like all men, was extremely vulnerable, and that to bolster him she had to show him great respect and to agree with his opinions.

At the beginning of analysis, Sylvia was threatened unconsciously by her sense of responsibility for the analyst. She feared that to protect him from being hurt, she would have to accept false interpretations or follow bad advice. Therefore, she planned at the beginning to work at disproving the pathogenic belief in her omnipotent responsibility for the analyst. The attainment of this goal was for her the precondition of getting involved in the treatment.

Sylvia worked unconsciously for many months to change her pathogenic belief by testing it in her relationship with the analyst. She tested it by disagreeing with him, hoping thereby to convince herself that she was not hurting him. She began this testing by tentatively questioning some of the analyst's opinions, while prepared to retract her questions if he gave evidence of being hurt. She was helped when she saw that the analyst was not upset by her questioning him, and so passed her tests. She was also helped by the analyst's interpreting her exaggerated sense of her power to hurt him. She became less afraid of hurting the analyst and thus more able to think critically about his comments.

As she acquired the capacity to disagree with the analyst, she permitted herself to confide in him and to become fond of him. Once she knew that she could reject his opinions, she felt safe feeling close to him. She also let herself feel closer to her husband.

This example illustrates a point about interpretation that has been demonstrated by quantitative research (see Chapter 8): A patient is especially helped by an interpretation that he can put to immediate use in his working to carry out his unconscious plans—that is, by a "pro-plan" interpretation. In the example above, the interpretation of the patient's exaggerated belief in her power to hurt the analyst was highly pro-plan. It was both true and of immediate use. It helped the patient both to become conscious of her pathogenic belief and to realize that the belief was false. Also, the fact that the analyst made the interpretation demonstrated that he was sympathetic with her wish to disprove the belief, and that he was able to help her do so.

The patient is set back by interpretations that hinder him in his efforts to carry out his plans—that is, by anti-plan interpretations. It seems likely that the patient presented above would have found the interpretation "You're afraid to trust me" highly anti-plan. She would have experienced it as confirming the belief that she must put blind faith in the analyst to avoid upsetting him.

A patient tests his pathogenic beliefs by experimental actions. He carries out an action that, according to his pathogenic belief, will affect the therapist in a particular way. The patient hopes unconsciously that this action will not affect the therapist as the belief predicts. If the patient's pathogenic expectation is not borne out, the patient may feel relieved and take a small step toward disconfirming the belief.

The patient may test his pathogenic beliefs verbally. For example, a patient who unconsciously believes that he will or should be punished for feeling proud may test this belief by a trial expression of pride. He hopes that the therapist will not put him down. Or a patient who unconsciously believes that he deserves to be rejected may test this belief by a trial expression of affection. He hopes that the therapist will not reject him by interpreting his affection as, for example, a defense against unconscious hostility.

A patient may also test his pathogenic beliefs by a trial change in nonverbal behavior. For example, a patient who unconsciously believes that he does not deserve treatment may test this belief by missing sessions. He hopes that the therapist will help him realize that he deserves to come to his sessions. Or a male patient who unconsciously believes that if he is friendly he will seduce his female therapist may test this belief by behaving seductively. He hopes that the therapist will demonstrate her nonseducibility.

In unconsciously planning his tests, the patient wishes to garner maximum evidence against his pathogenic beliefs at minimum risk. In some instances the patient, by careful unconscious planning, is able to test his pathogenic beliefs gradually in a series of graded tests, none of which puts him at much risk. In other instances the patient is unable to work at a safe rate. This was true of a patient who suffered such severe survivor guilt at the beginning of treatment that she could not commit herself to treatment until she had given, and the therapist had passed, a dangerous test: She provided the therapist with considerable (albeit false) evidence that she was so disturbed that she was untreatable. She was able to let herself become a patient only after the therapist had demonstrated that he was not deterred by her damaging self-accusations and that he did not take them at face value (see Modell, 1965).

The patient may test his pathogenic beliefs in two different ways: namely, by turning passive into active, and by transferring. In both kinds of tests the patient re-enacts the childhood traumatic experiences from which he inferred his pathogenic beliefs. In passive-into-active testing, the patient behaves to the therapist in the traumatic ways that a parent behaved toward him. The patient hopes to demonstrate that the therapist will not be upset by him as he was by his parents. He does not want the therapist to be constrained by pathogenic beliefs such as those from which he himself suffers. If the patient infers that the therapist is not upset, he may be relieved. He may observe the therapist dealing effectively with behavior that was for him traumatic, and so may learn from the therapist how to deal effectively with such behavior. This is illustrated by the case of Andrea M., discussed below.

Andrea M.

Andrea M. came to therapy in her late 20s. She had been traumatized in childhood by her parents' depressions, weaknesses, and vulnerabilities. Her parents had needed her to appreciate them, to depend on them, and to agree with them. If she did not they would accuse her of being selfish, and would become upset, pout, and complain. They were still behaving this way at the time the patient began her therapy.

Andrea complied with the belief that she was responsible for her parents' unhappiness. She tried to keep them happy by remaining their adoring, servile daughter. However, she did not succeed in buoying them up, and she accepted the implied accusation that she was a selfish, worthless person.

During the first phase of treatment, Andrea tried to keep the therapist happy. After about 6 months she began to test the therapist by turning passive into active; she began to treat the therapist as her parents had treated her. She would imply overwhelming disappointment in the therapist if she experienced him as failing to show her the utmost respect. She would feel insulted by comments the therapist clearly intended as benign, and she would become highly indignant if the therapist came a minute late. She would tell the therapist that he was being horrible, ruining her relationship with him, and making treatment almost impossible.

The therapist tried to pass Andrea's tests by remaining concerned about her while not accepting her blame. Sometimes he would respond to her criticisms by saying nothing. At other times he would attempt to draw her out about her complaining, and at still other times he would try to make her aware that she was afraid she was hurting him. Also, he would occasionally tell her that she was trying to show him by her behavior how her parents had treated her.

Andrea's reactions to the therapist depended, among other factors, on her inferences about how her complaining was affecting him. When she inferred that she was upsetting him, she would become more depressed and more vituperative in her blame. When she inferred that she was not upsetting him, she would become stronger, less depressed, and in some instances more insightful. She would think about her complaining; she would then begin to realize that she felt guilty about it, and that she was behaving as her parents had behaved.

By her passive-into-active testing, Andrea was attempting to find out whether in his relationship with her the therapist was guided by pathogenic beliefs similar to those that guided her in her relationship with her parents. She hoped to assure herself that he was not like her; that he did not feel omnipotently responsible for her happiness; and that he did not feel like a bad person, even though he sometimes was unable to help her.

Gradually, over a period of time, Andrea gained the assurance she sought. She identified with the therapist's capacity not to feel bad when she blamed him. As she did so, she modified her pathogenic belief that she had to comply with her parents' blame. She became more conscious of this belief and of the experiences from which she had inferred it. She became more conscious, too, that she had suffered from her belief in her omnipotent responsibility for her parents, and that she had been behaving toward the therapist as her parents had behaved toward her.

A patient may test his pathogenic beliefs more directly by transference tests than by passive-into-active tests. In transference tests, he behaves with the therapist as in childhood he behaved with his parents. He reproduces the behavior that, in his opinion, provoked the parental reactions from which he inferred his pathogenic beliefs. The patient unconsciously hopes that he will not affect the therapist as he affected his parents. He may hope, for example, that he will not, by his sexuality, provoke the therapist to punish him, or by his contentment provoke the therapist to charge him with complacency, or by his independence cause the therapist to feel rejected. If the patient observes that he does not affect the therapist as he affected a parent, he may take a step toward disconfirming the belief that he provoked the traumatic parental reactions.

Andrea M. (Continued)

As Andrea became less convinced of her responsibility for others and less vulnerable to blame from them, she could risk letting herself feel fond of them. In the therapy, while continuing to test the therapist by turning passive into active, she also began to test him by transferring. She tested him by trial expressions of fondness, in the hope that the therapist would permit her to like him; she also tested him by accusing herself of being selfish, destructive, and unworthy, in the hope that he would disagree.

As the therapist passed these tests, Andrea made further progress. She established a still better relationship with the therapist, which enabled her to realize more directly that she had not been the cause of her parents' unhappiness and that she was not a disagreeable selfish person.

All patients test the therapist throughout therapy, both by turning passive into active and by transferring. Often the patient gives both kinds of tests simultaneously by the same behavior. Consider, for example, a patient whose parents blamed him frequently for minor offenses and who by identifying with them did the same to them and to others. By blaming the therapist, the patient may be putting himself in the role of his parents, hoping to discover that he does not hurt the therapist by his blame as his parents hurt him. However, he may also be putting the therapist in the role of his parents, hoping to demonstrate that the therapist will not be provoked by his blame as his parents were provoked by it.

In some therapies the patient is comfortable giving transference tests from the beginning. In other therapies the patient may feel safer giving passive-into-active tests in the beginning, because while turning passive into active the patient is putting himself in the strong position of the aggressor, and thereby providing himself with a defense against being traumatized by the therapist. In still other therapies the patient at the beginning unconsciously considers it dangerous to turn passive into active. He may fear that he will traumatize the therapist so severely that he will render the therapist unable to help him; or he may realize how much he was hurt by his parents' behavior, and so may fear that he would feel intense guilt if he were to behave with the therapist as his parents behaved with him.

TECHNIQUE

The theory of technique proposed here follows from the formulations presented above. It assumes that the therapist's basic task is to offer the patient the help he seeks in his struggle to change his pathogenic beliefs and to pursue the goals they warn him against. The therapist, by his overall approach, his attitude, his reactions to the patient's tests, and his interpretations, helps the patient to feel safe and secure with him. He thereby helps the patient to face the dangers predicted by his pathogenic beliefs, and to work at the task of disconfirming them.

The recommendation that the therapist help the patient to feel safe and secure contrasts with the recommendation of Freud in his 1911–1915 theory that the therapist be neutral. Consider the case of the patient who suffers from the unconscious pathogenic belief that he will and should be rejected by the therapist. According to the 1911–1915 theory, the therapist should be neutral with the patient. If he is friendly and accepting, he may gratify the patient's unconscious dependency, and thus make it more difficult for the patient to realize that he fears that the therapist will reject him. In contrast, the theory proposed here assumes that when the patient feels reassured against the danger of rejection, he may feel safe enough to face his fear that the therapist will reject him. (For quantitative research comparing the explanatory power of the two theories, see Chapter 8.)

The means the therapist may use to help a patient feel safe and secure depend on the nature of the patient's pathogenic beliefs. The therapist's approach is case-specific. His techniques are geared to helping the patient feel reassured against the dangers predicted by his particular pathogenic beliefs, and to work at disproving these beliefs in accordance with his own plans for doing so.

The Relation of the Present Theory to Freud's Ego Psychology

The present theory contrasts clearly with Freud's early theory of the mind. In the latter, which may be referred to as based on the "automatic-functioning hypothesis" (AFH), the mind consists of psychic forces—namely, impulses and defenses—that are regulated "automatically" (Freud, 1900, p. 600; 1905, p. 266) by the pleasure principle without regard for thoughts, plans, or beliefs. The impulses continually seek their gratifications, and the defenses oppose the impulses' coming forth. From the dynamic interactions of the impulses and defenses are derived almost all of the phenomena of psychic life (Freud, 1926b, p. 255).

The patient, according to the 1911–1915 theory, has no unconscious wish to solve his problems; indeed, he continually resists the therapy. The therapist tries to help the patient by analyzing his resistances. His ultimate goal is to help the patient to make the unconscious conscious. By doing this, he enables the patient to gain control of the previously repressed infantile impulses and to redirect them to mature purposes.

Certain concepts scattered in passages throughout Freud's late works are the starting point for the present theory. These concepts assume the patient's capacity to make use unconsciously of higher mental functions, and so may be referred to as constituting the "higher-mental-functioning hypothesis" (HMFH). In parts of his late theory, Freud assumed that a person may suffer unconsciously from a pathogenic belief (e.g., the belief in castration as a punishment). There Freud assumed, too, that a person exerts some control over his repressions (1940a, p. 199), and that he can unconsciously think, test reality, and make and carry out decisions and plans (1940a, p. 199). He postulated a powerful unconscious wish to solve problems (1920, pp. 32, 35; 1926a, p. 167), and he assumed that the patient may work with the therapist to master his problems (1937, p. 35).

Despite the development by Freud of the ideas presented above, the psychoanalytic theory of technique, in its various versions, is still based largely on Freud's early theory of the mind (Lipton, 1967, p. 91; Coltrera & Ross, 1967, p. 38; Kanzer & Blum, 1967, pp. 138–139; Weinshel, 1970). There are several reasons for this: The big advances in Freud's theorizing cited above are contained in isolated passages in his later works, often in discussions of basic theory. They have not been systematically applied to the understanding of therapy and technique. Moreover, the 1911–1915 theory was so systematically developed and so widely accepted by analysts that technical ideas based on the HMFH were simply added onto this theory; no organic changes were made in it. Thus, most present-day versions of the psychoanalytic theory of technique are in essence modifications of the 1911–1915 theory. They contain concepts from ego psychology that can be assimilated to the 1911–1915 theory without fundamentally changing it.

In contrast, the theory proposed here is built from the ground up on the HMFH of Freud's late writings.

A Schematic Comparison of the 1911–1915 Theory of Technique with the Theory Proposed Here

The assumptions of the 1911–1915 theory may be put schematically as follows:

1. The patient's symptoms and character defects are maintained as a consequence of the gratifications that the patient unconsciously attains from the fixation of certain of his impulses to infantile objects and aims.

2. The patient's most powerful unconscious motive is to retain such gratifications and thus to retain his psychopathology. Indeed, the patient has no unconscious wish to make progress; rather, he is strongly motivated to resist the therapist's attempts to help him, lest he be forced to relinquish the infantile gratifications.

3. The unconscious repetitions in the transference of childhood experiences are regulated beyond the patient's control by the pleasure principle and the repetition compulsion. These repetitions are intended unconsciously either to provide gratifications in relation to the therapist, or, by serving as transference resistances, to protect the unconscious gratifications that the patient obtains in his psychopathology.

The theory of therapy on which my views of technique are based contrasts with each of the propositions of the 1911–1915 theory as outlined above. It assumes the following:

1. The patient's symptoms and character problems are maintained by pathogenic beliefs that are developed in early childhood by inference from experience. These beliefs warn the patient that if he relinquishes his psychopathology, he may put himself or his loved ones in danger.

2. The patient is powerfully motivated unconsciously to make progress but is afraid to do so, lest he put himself or someone he loves in danger. His anxiety about moving forward stems from his pathogenic beliefs and from the feelings of danger to which they give rise.

3. The various repetitions in the transference of the patient's childhood experiences are unconsciously purposeful. They are brought about by the patient for various purposes, one of which is to test his pathogenic beliefs.

The two theories point the therapist's attention in different directions. A therapist who is guided by the 1911–1915 theory asks himself, "What are the patient's major defenses and resistances? What unconscious impulses, including transferences, are seeking expression? How may I best frustrate these impulses, as a step toward making them conscious? What resistances and what impulses should I interpret?"

In contrast, the therapist guided by the theory presented here asks himself, "What are the patient's pathogenic beliefs? How is he working to change them? What are his current goals and plans? How is he testing me? How may I make it safer for him to carry out his plans and thus to reach his goals? How may I best pass the patient's tests? What interpretations may help him to reach his goals?"

DISTINCTIVE FEATURES OF THE PRESENT THEORY

The Theory Is Highly Empirical

I developed the basic concepts of the present theory by studying the process notes of long segments of the analyses of a number of patients. My purpose was to learn how patients change. Since the theory was developed through careful scrutiny of clinical material, its concepts are close to observation and may readily be tested empirically. They may be tested informally by the clinician, and formally by quantitative research studies.

The theory may readily be expanded by empirical methods. For example, my colleagues and I have demonstrated in numerous formal research studies that the patient feels less endangered, more relaxed, and more insightful immediately after the therapist passes a significant test or makes a pro-plan interpretation. Having established that patients become less endangered when the therapist is helpful, we have been able to discover various ways in which patients are endangered and various ways in which therapists may help them. For example, from observing my patients' reactions to my interventions, I became convinced that certain patients during the opening months of therapy are endangered by any interpretation, and that such patients may respond favorably only when the therapist refrains from interpreting.

The present theory has been tested by the Mount Zion Psychotherapy Research Group for over 20 years, using formal quantitative research methods. The research is reported in Chapter 8. In these studies we have found strong support for the idea that the patient exerts control over his unconscious mental life. He keeps mental contents repressed as long as he unconsciously assumes that they are dangerous, and permits them to come forth when he unconsciously decides that he may safely do so. We have also found strong support for the ideas that the patient suffers from pathogenic beliefs; that in therapy he develops plans for disproving these beliefs; and that he works throughout therapy by testing these beliefs with the therapist in order to disprove them. Other investigators, including Horowitz (1991), Horowitz & Stinson (1991), Luborsky (1988), Dahl (1980) and Dahl, Kächele, and Thomä (1988), have also studied the pertinence of higher mental functioning in unconscious mental life.

The Patient Is Almost Always Working to Get Better

Much of the patient's behavior—including behavior in which the patient appears bored, insulting, or grossly uncooperative —is part of the patient's working, both consciously and unconsciously, to get better. Even when the patient is unable unconsciously to control his behavior, as when he gives in to guilt and becomes selfdestructive, he may secondarily observe the therapist to determine whether the therapist approves of or opposes his selfdestructiveness.

A patient who is uncooperative may be testing the therapist by turning passive into active. That is, he may be behaving toward the therapist as in his experience a parent behaved toward him. The patient hopes that he will not discourage or crush the therapist as he himself was discouraged or crushed by the parental behavior. If a therapist passes the patient's tests by not reacting as the patient reacted to the traumatizing parental behavior, the patient may feel better. Then he may use the therapist as a model to fight the parental attitudes that he has internalized.

The Patient Sets the Agenda

The patient rather than the therapist sets the agenda. The patient conveys to the therapist, albeit at times indirectly, how he would like to work in therapy. He permits the therapist to infer the goals he would like to pursue and the pathogenic beliefs that prevent him from pursuing these goals (see Chapter 4). The therapist's task, then, is to help the patient, in accordance with the patient's unconscious plans, to disprove his pathogenic beliefs and to pursue his goals. The therapist may learn whether or not he is passing the patient's tests or making helpful (proplan) interpretations by observing the patient's reactions to him. If the therapist is on the right track, the patient will become bolder and more insightful. Then in some instances, after a brief period of relief, the patient may develop the courage to test his pathogenic beliefs more vigorously. If the therapist is on the wrong track, the patient will become more timid, more depressed, and less insightful, and he may test his pathogenic beliefs less vigorously.

No Non-Case-Specific Set of Technical Rules is Sufficient to Offer Optimal Help to the Patient

The patient uses his considerable unconscious capacity for inference to infer as accurately as he can just what the therapist intends by his attitudes, interventions, and interpretations. The patient is especially concerned with discerning the therapist's attitudes toward his pathogenic beliefs and plans. The therapist may offer optimal help to the patient only if he infers the patient's plans and helps him to carry them out by passing the patient's tests and by giving him pro-plan interpretations.

If the therapist is guided in his behavior by a set of non-case-specific technical rules, no matter how subtle these may be, he is unlikely to pass all of the patient's tests unless he is in fact sympathetic to the patient's plans. This is because the patient unconsciously will see around the rules and infer the therapist's attitude to his plans. Nonetheless, certain patients, because of their considerable ability unconsciously to infer the therapist's intentions, may be helped (if not optimally) by a therapist who is guided by a certain set of technical rules. Such a patient, by inferring the therapist's rules, may know just how the therapist is likely to react to him, and he will use this knowledge to devise tests that the therapist is likely to pass.

Powerful Maladaptive Impulses Are Held in Place by Pathogenic Beliefs

The present theory differs from the 1911–1915 theory in that Freud assumed that maladaptive behavior stems ultimately from powerful unconscious infantile impulses, such as greed, lust, hatred, envy, and so forth. According to the present theory, explanations in terms of powerful maladaptive impulses are never fundamental, for such impulses are invariably held in place by pathogenic beliefs.

For example, a patient to be described in Chapter 2 expressed almost uncontrollable sexual passion. She was motivated by guilt about feeling that she was better than her mother. The patient was proud of her chastity but felt guilty about being superior to her mother, who had been highly promiscuous. She punished herself for feeling superior to her mother by feeling out of control of her sexuality. She gained control of her sexuality when she was helped by the therapist to realize that she was tormenting herself with it so as not to feel superior to her mother.

The Therapist Should Attempt to Help the Patient Reconstruct the Traumatic Experiences from Which the Patient Inferred His Pathogenic Beliefs

The present theory disagrees with those theoreticians who recommend that the therapist focus primarily on the impulses and affects that the patient expresses to the therapist in the here and now, and that he be concerned only secondarily (if at all), with the reconstruction of the patient's childhood traumatic experiences.

The reconstruction of the childhood traumas is of great importance. Unless the therapist knows how the patient acquired his problems, the therapist cannot know the patient's pathogenic beliefs, or his goals, or how to pass his tests. A patient may express a particular impulse to the therapist for a variety of reasons, and unless the therapist knows why the patient is expressing it, he will not know how to deal with it. For example, a patient may have developed a tendency in childhood to express maladaptive anger and hostility because he inferred that by being unreasonably angry, he permitted his mother to feel morally superior to him. Another patient may have developed a tendency to hostility and negativism as part of a struggle to fight off compliance to a parent who abused him. The two patients, by expressing hostility to the therapist, are giving him different kinds of tests. The patient who became enraged to please his mother attempts by his display of anger to assure himself that the therapist is not motivated to feel morally superior to him. This patient wishes to convince himself that the therapist wants him to be reasonable and controlled. The patient who is angry in order to fight off compliance attempts by his display of hostility and negativism to assure himself that the therapist does not object to his hostility. He wants to convince himself that the therapist will not deprive him of a tool he needs to protect himself from being abused. Such a patient may be unwilling to relinquish his anger until he knows the therapist can comfortably tolerate it.

The Corrective Emotional Experience

The present theory assumes that the patient seeks corrective emotional experiences through his testing, and that the therapist should provide the patient with the experiences he seeks. The idea of offering the patient a corrective emotional experience makes no sense in the theory proposed by Freud in the *Papers on Technique*. In the 1911–1915 theory, the patient's unconscious mind consists solely of impulses and defenses, not of beliefs that may be disproved by experience. However, the idea of offering the patient corrective emotional experiences does fit with the present theory. Because psychopathology stems primarily from unconscious maladaptive beliefs, the patient, by testing the therapist throughout therapy, seeks experiences with the therapist that he may use in his efforts to disprove these beliefs. Moreover, as our research has demonstrated, the patient benefits when the therapist helps the patient to obtain the experiences he seeks.

The therapist who attempts to pass the patient's tests by offering the patient the experiences he seeks need not fear that he will go far astray, for, as already noted, he may check the pertinence of his behavior to the patient by the patient's reactions to him.

CHAPTER 2

Affect, Motivation, and Adaptation

This chapter continues my presentation of basic theory. It develops the thesis, introduced in Chapter 1, that beginning in infancy a person works throughout life to understand his reality and adapt to it. As part of this effort, he seeks reliable knowledge (beliefs) about himself and his interpersonal world, and also about the moral and ethical assumptions of this world. Whether normal or pathogenic, these beliefs are central to his conscious and unconscious mental life.

This conceptualization indicates that in order to understand the patient, the therapist should infer the patient's conscious and unconscious beliefs about himself and his interpersonal world. The therapist may then perceive the patient's situation, with its dangers and its opportunities, much as the patient himself perceives it. The therapist may thus come to understand how to help the patient to deal with the dangers and to take advantage of the opportunities.

THE CONCEPT OF REALITY IN FREUD'S EARLY AND LATE THEORIZING

In his early writings Freud minimized a person's unconscious concern for reality. He assumed that in infancy a person is narcissistic, and that he becomes interested in reality only as a consequence of hard experience (Freud, 1900). Moreover,

Freud assumed that throughout life a person is unconsciously motivated by powerful impulses. These are close to instinct,[1] unaffected by reality, and regulated by the pleasure principle.

However, in his late writings Freud credited a person with a strong unconscious wish to adapt to reality. Freud derived this wish from the task of self-preservation (1940a, p. 199). A person carrying out this task tests reality (p. 199), regulates his behavior unconsciously by the criteria of safety and danger (p. 199), and strives to gain control over the demands of his instincts (p. 144).

A number of analysts since Freud, beginning with Hartmann (1939, 1956a, 1956b), have discussed the importance in a person's mental life of the struggle to adapt to reality. Hartmann wrote that a person becomes adapted to reality not simply as a consequence of hard experience but also through a capacity (independent of the drives) for anticipation and postponement, and through an independent motivation toward adaptation. In Hartmann's words, "Something in the person speaks out for reality" (1956a, p. 243).

The formulations of Freud cited above, and those of Hartmann and others, have not been applied systematically at the clinical level. Thus many psychoanalysts and many psychotherapists of various persuasions, including those who emphasize the importance of object relations in development, base their clinical thinking on the theory presented by Freud in his early writings. These therapists assume that powerful manifestations of sex and aggression, such as urgent sexual interests, rage, jealousy, and envy, are selfish (narcissistic) infantilisms un-

---

[1]In his early writings Freud assumed that unconscious instinctual impulses are ultimately sexual—that is, that they are derived from and express sexual instincts. Later he assumed that they may be derived from sexual or aggressive instincts or some combination of these.

Stern (1985, p. 238) has written that his direct observations of infants do not support the idea of one or two basic instincts. According to Stern, motivation needs to be reconceptualized as organized by interrelated systems that unfold developmentally. These are classified as "ego instincts," and they include attachment (to parents), exploration, curiosity, certain perceptual preferences, cognitive novelty, and pleasure in mastery. For a comprehensive discussion of motivation somewhat similar to Stern's, see Lichtenberg (1989).

touched by reality and regulated primarily by the pleasure principle. They do not share my assumption that these motives, affects, and behaviors express not only inborn impulses, but also attempts to adapt to reality as it is perceived or believed to be.

THE EMPIRICAL STUDIES OF DANIEL STERN

The idea that the infant or young child is intensely interested in understanding his reality is supported by the research of Daniel Stern (1985) and others (Brazelton & Yogman, 1989; Emde, 1989). According to Stern (whose research does not support the idea of a primitive stage of narcissism or of autism), the infant begins learning about his reality at birth. For example, he learns after 3 days to recognize his mother's milk by its smell (1985, p. 39), and after several weeks to recognize her voice. The infant regulates his behavior according to his beliefs about reality and not in accordance with fantasy. Thus Stern writes that "infants . . . are concerned with events that actually happened. . . . there are no wish fulfilling fantasies. The infant is thus seen as an excellent reality tester. . . . reality at this stage is never distorted for defensive reasons" (1985, p. 11). Also, in agreement with Bruner (1977), Stern writes, "From birth on there appears to be a central tendency to form and test hypotheses about what is happening in the world" (1985, p. 42). Finally, Stern writes that "infants from the beginning mainly experience reality. Their subjective experiences suffer no distortion by virtue of wishes or defenses, but only those made inevitable by perceptual or cognitive immaturity or overgeneralization" (p. 255).

As regards the relative importance in the mental life of the infant of the pleasure principle and the reality principle, Stern writes:

> It seems apparent that the ability of infants to deal with reality has to be considered on a par with the ability to deal with hedonics and that ego formation is better differentiated and functioning than Glover or Hartmann could have known. Further-

more, many of the corollaries that flowed from the basic assumption of id before ego, such as the idea that the primary process (autistic) thinking precedes secondary process (reality or socialized) thinking, were also arbitrary. (1985, pp. 239–240)

A PERSON'S FIRST EFFORTS AT ADAPTATION

The first reality that a person faces is that of himself, his parents, and his siblings. He makes his first efforts to adapt, and acquires his first knowledge of himself and others, in relation to them. Since the infant or young child is completely dependent on his parents, his only good strategy for adaptation is to develop a reasonable working relationship with them; that is, he seeks a relationship in which he is firmly connected to them and can rely on them to meet his needs for care. His maintaining his ties to his parents is so important to him that he does whatever he believes he must do to accomplish this. He is powerfully motivated to comply with whatever he believes would please his parents, including behavior that manifestly is not pleasing.

For example, a boy of 5 was "bad" in relation to his father, not from primary anger, hostility, or defiance, but as part of an effort to maintain his all-important ties to him. The boy's father was depressed, irritable, and noncommunicative. However, the father would come to life when reprimanding the boy for being messy or noisy. The boy inferred from this and from his father's failure to praise him when he was neat and quiet that his father was more interested in exerting parental authority over him than in helping him. Thus, by being noisy and messy, the boy was offering his father opportunities to exert parental authority. He hoped that by doing this he would please his father and maintain a connection with him.

In the following example, a 6-year-old boy, Alex N., was "bad" and uncooperative as part of an active and adaptive effort to induce a parent to be the authority he needed in order to feel secure. Alex was frightened by his power to dominate his father, and he succeeded by his provocative behavior in getting his father to demonstrate a sense of authority.

Alex N.

Alex was a highly intelligent, outgoing child whose fond father was eager to teach him to be a good sport. The boy professed interest in playing games with his father, but would become provocative when his father tried to play with him. For example, his father would set up a board game and Alex would knock it down. His father, who hoped by example to teach Alex patience, would carefully prepare the board again, and the boy would knock it over again.

As Alex continued his provocative behavior, his father became genuinely baffled and consulted a child psychotherapist who was a friend of the family. The therapist told the father, "You and your son are working at cross purposes. Your priority is to teach your son good sportsmanship. His is to induce you to exert more authority with him, be less worried about him, and take his whims less seriously. You should do this. He feels anxious and unprotected, and is trying to get you to change."

As the father put his friend's advice into practice, his son became calmer and less provocative. After several months the boy, whose father was now taking more authority, began to enjoy playing games with his father.

A child as young as 18 months whose mother is depressed may attempt to cheer her up as part of his effort to obtain from her the care he needs (Zahn-Waxler & Radke-Yarrow, 1982). He may do so by being cheerful and excited, or even by hitting his mother or being provocatively disobedient.

OTHER ASPECTS OF ADAPTATION IN THE PRESENT THEORY

To Adapt, a Person Must Learn the Moral Assumptions of His World

Among the important parts of a person's reality are the moral and ethical assumptions (beliefs) that others expect him to follow in his relations with them, and that guide them in their relations with him. A person who settles in an unfamiliar culture soon learns that the moral and ethical assumptions of that culture are part of his new reality, and that to adapt to this culture he must learn them and abide by them. This applies even more strongly to the infant or young child in relation to his family: In order to adapt, he must learn the moral and ethical assumptions that guide his parents. These assumptions are an important part of his reality; if he does not learn them, he risks censure, humiliation, and punishment.

The infant or young child does not conceive of morality as a separate and distinct part of reality. Nor does he learn his moral ideas separately from the rest of his ideas about reality. Rather, he endows all important interactions with his parents with what, from the adults' point of view, is moral significance. He assumes that the ways his parents treat him are the ways he should be treated; in other words, he endows his parents' judgments of him with both real and moral meanings. For example, the judgment that he is bad is for him not different in kind from the judgment that he is stupid. Each judgment is for him both real and moral. If the infant or child did not assume that the ways his parents treat him are the ways he should be treated, he would not develop a superego that, as Freud wrote, "observes the ego, gives it orders, judges it and threatens it with punishments, exactly like the parents whose place it has taken" (1940a, p. 205).

My formulations and reconstructions from adult analyses support the idea that whether a child becomes guilty to his parents depends mainly on how his parents react to him. He does not develop feelings of guilt about his hostility to his parents unless he infers from observation, or is told by his parents, that by being hostile to them he hurts them. On the other hand, the child who is not hostile to his parents may become guilty to them if they complain that he is upsetting them. Moreover, since the child tends to take responsibility for his parents' behavior, he may, even if not hostile, become guilty to them if they are unhappy, withdrawn, or rejecting. The child then may secondarily become angry at his parents for making him feel guilty. Also, he may confuse cause and effect, and so come to believe that he feels guilty *because* he is angry (Settlage, personal communication, 1989).

In one case a male patient, whose childhood had been marred by an extremely abusive mother, demonstrated his sense of responsibility for her behavior by his persistent and vigorous efforts to disavow this responsibility. The patient complained hour after hour in a monotonous way about the harmful things his mother had done to him, until the therapist, who had good reason to believe the patient, assured him that he (the therapist) believed the patient's account of his mother's behavior; in addition, he believed that the patient had not provoked it. The therapist also told the patient that he seemed to be struggling against a tendency to blame himself unfairly for how his mother had treated him. After this, the patient gradually stopped his complaining about his mother and began to become aware that he had indeed previously believed in his responsibility for his mother's bad behavior.

It Is Adaptive for a Person Not to Change Beliefs about Reality Too Rapidly

Ordinarily the adult, and to a lesser extent the child, is slow to change his conscious and unconscious beliefs about himself and his interpersonal world. When exposed to experiences that run counter to his beliefs, he is likely to assimilate the experiences to the beliefs. For example, a student who suffers from the belief that he is weak in academic skills may discount his doing well on an exam by assuming that he was lucky, or that the exam was easy, or that the teacher was lax in grading it.

In his tendency to retain his beliefs about reality, a person in everyday life behaves like a scientist who, having understood his field in terms of his theories, tends to retain the theories, unless forced by striking new evidence to change them. Like the scientist, the person in everyday life tends to weigh evidence that confirms his beliefs more heavily than evidence that runs counter to them. This is adaptive. Neither the person in everyday life nor the scientist in his research could function if he were to change his basic beliefs with each new experience. Both need a relatively stable set of beliefs to guide them in their attempts to make and carry out their plans. Even a relatively poor guide may be better than a constantly changing one.

This principle applies to both normal and pathogenic beliefs. Additional factors hold for pathogenic beliefs. A person is especially motivated both to retain such beliefs and to change them. He is especially motivated to change a pathogenic belief because he suffers from it; however, he fears that if he does so he will experience the dangers that the belief warns him against. Consider, for example, an exaggeratedly altruistic patient who suffered from the belief that if he became more selfish he would hurt others. Since he suffered from having to be so altruistic, he was highly motivated to change this belief. However, he was quite reluctant to test it for fear of hurting others.

Beliefs Are More Fundamental than Fantasies

A person's beliefs about reality are a more fundamental part of his personality than are his wishful fantasies. In infancy a person does not permit himself to escape reality by denial or by wishful fantasy. When in childhood he begins to permit denial or fantasy, he does so in relation to a pre-existing understanding of reality. For example, a person does not develop a wishful fantasy of having great power unless he believes that he has little or no power. Nor does a boy develop the fantasy that women possess penises unless he believes that women are supposed to have penises but have lost them by castration.

A person regulates his use of denial or of fantasy not in accordance with the pleasure principle (as in Freud's early theory), but in accordance with his unconscious assessments of reality. Ordinarily he considers it more adaptive to remain oriented to reality. However, in certain circumstances he may consider it more adaptive to escape reality by use of denial or by fantasy:

1. He may in certain circumstances unconsciously decide that facing a certain frightening reality is more dangerous than denying it. For example, he may assume that if he faced a certain horrifying reality, he would become so upset that he could not act to protect himself from danger.

2. He may decide that he is helpless to affect his fate and thus that he has nothing to lose by denial. For example, during their internments, some prisoners of war in Vietnam permitted

themselves blissful wish fulfillment dreams only after becoming convinced that they could do nothing to improve their situations (Balson, 1975). At that point their blissful dreams were adaptive. In their dreams the helpless prisoners defied the guards who had been tormenting them, offered themselves a measure of hope in a situation of despair, and helped themselves to enjoy much-needed restful sleep. (See Chapter 7 for a further discussion of blissful dreams.)

3. He may unconsciously decide that he is so safe that he would not endanger himself by turning from reality. For example, an adult may decide this while on vacation, or a child when he feels especially protected by his parents.

A person may turn from his reality as a consequence of his pathogenic beliefs about himself and his world. For example, he may do this if he unconsciously believes that he lives in such a hostile world and is so weak that he cannot protect himself (see Chapter 7). Or, he may do this out of loyalty to a parent or sibling who is himself unable to face his reality.

A Person Assesses His Reality by His Affective Responses to It

A person, in assessing his reality and deciding how he should react to it, takes account not only of his thoughts about it, but also (and often primarily) of his affective responses to it. A person's affective responses are based on certain conscious and unconscious inferences about reality and may be adaptive. A person may respond affectively to his reality in a prompt and decisive manner even before he can assess it by conscious verbal thought. For example, as a consequence of his affective responses to a particular salesman, a buyer may begin to consider the possibility that the salesman is cheating him before he can figure this out by conscious thought.

The idea that a patient's affective responses to his reality provide him with information (however subjective) about it helps explain the value of his becoming conscious of his repressed affects. A person, by becoming conscious of his repressed affective responses to another person, may learn a great deal about his relationship to that person. For example, an analytic patient first became aware that his childhood relations to his parents had been unsatisfactory by becoming conscious of his intense anger to them. He began to realize that he had often felt humiliated by his mother, whom he perceived as competitive, and that he had felt chronically rejected by his father, whom he perceived as withdrawn and self-centered. These realizations permitted the patient to become conscious of a pathogenic belief in his inadequacy that he inferred from his mother's derision, and of a pathogenic belief that he was uninteresting that he inferred from his father's indifference.

A Person's Personality Reflects His Attempts at Adaptation

The idea that a person may organize his affects, impulses, behaviors, and goals in accordance with his reality is obvious in certain dramatic situations—for instance, when he has been offered a coveted award, or when he has received news of the death of a beloved child, or when his marriage proposal has been accepted by the woman he loves. In such situations, a person's immediate reality is so powerful that it is likely to override the realities that his conscious and unconscious beliefs portray for him. However, even in such dramatic circumstances, a person's feelings and behavior may diverge from the expected; his perceptions of his situation may be based on certain highly personal conscious and unconscious beliefs that depict a reality different from his reality as assessed by an observer. For example, the man whose proposal has just been accepted may be quite unhappy, for one of a number of reasons: He may believe that nothing he does can work out, or that all women are untrustworthy, or that he cannot or should not be happier in his marriage than his parents were in theirs.

In situations in which a person's reality is not compelling, he organizes his affects, impulses, goals, and behaviors, and perceives himself and his interpersonal world, primarily in accordance with his conscious and unconscious beliefs about reality. Thus, as a consequence of these beliefs a person may characteristically feel weak or strong, intelligent or stupid, deserving or undeserving. He may be optimistic or pessimistic, cheerful or dour, brave or cowardly, careful or careless, trusting or suspicious. He may be ambitious or unambitious, proud or ashamed, stubborn or yielding, cooperative or uncooperative, and so forth.

Powerful, Urgent Maladaptive Impulses Reflect Adaptation to a Maladaptive (Pathogenic) Picture of Reality

Freud's early theory and the theory proposed here provide different explanations for the urgency of certain maladaptive impulses. In Freud's early theory, this urgency stems from the power of the pleasure principle and is fueled by sexual and aggressive energy. In the theory proposed here, this urgency stems only secondarily from instinct. It stems primarily from the patient's pathogenic beliefs about reality and morality; such beliefs may have an awesome authority.

Thus, powerful maladaptive impulses may be maintained by pathogenic beliefs that are developed in infancy or early childhood in an attempt at adaptation. An infant or child may develop such beliefs in order to maintain his ties to his parents. For example, as already pointed out, a patient may become maladaptively "bad" if he infers that by being so he pleases a parent by giving the parent an opportunity to feel morally superior to him. Moreover, he may generalize this belief, and so may continue for years to behave provocatively with parent surrogates in an unconscious attempt to maintain his ties to them.

A person's maladaptive belief in his omnipotent responsibility for others may underlie his maladaptive urgent sexual behavior. Consider, for example, a 25-year-old woman who was sexually attracted to weak, critical, and judgmental men. Her interest in these men was based on beliefs inferred from her relationship with her unhappy, judgmental father, that by rejecting this type of man she might destroy him, and that by loving him she might restore him. In her family, her role had been to pacify her angry father by being docile, flattering, and attractive to him, and by agreeing with his angry outbursts.

After leaving home she maintained sexual alliances with weak, difficult men in an attempt to bolster them. She had great trouble leaving the man with whom she was having an unhappy affair; she assumed that if she rejected him he would become inconsolable and perhaps suicidal.

As therapy helped her to take her own needs more seriously, she began to pull away from this inadequate man. However, when he asked her to have intercourse without protection and so to risk becoming pregnant, she experienced an overwhelming desire to comply. She told her therapist that she was overwhelmed by her sexual desire. When her therapist suggested that her primary motivation was to make her boyfriend feel powerful, she readily agreed. She realized that the sense of urgency that she had assumed to be based on a sexual impulse was in fact based on a powerful wish to restore her boyfriend.

In certain of the examples presented below, the patients developed and maintained intense impulses as a consequence of survivor guilt. In these instances the patients' impulses appeared strong, not because they were derived from powerful instincts, but because they were fueled by the patients' consciences. The patients used the impulses to punish themselves. Thus these impulses expressed not powerful instinctual urges, but guilt derived from pathogenic beliefs.

In the first of these examples, a patient who suffered from survivor guilt developed a powerful "daemonic" sexual urge out of loyalty to her mother.

Talia S.

Talia S., a lawyer aged 39, grew up in dire poverty; she was raised by her mother and aunt, who were immigrants. They were severe alcoholics, neglectful, and dissolute. During her childhood her mother would conduct sexual orgies outside her bedroom. Her aunt on occasion would become drunk and stagger around the house, brandishing a knife and threatening to kill the patient.

Talia married, was divorced, and had one child by the age of 19. Her husband was unstable and abusive.

Talia's character was shaped by her struggle to escape the

sordid life of her childhood and adolescence. After taking much abuse, she learned to fight back; she made up her mind not to be taken advantage of. She became ambitious, obtained scholarships to college and law school, did well academically, graduated, and found a job as a public defender.

When Talia was 36, she converted to a strict fundamentalist religious sect. She attended church daily and adhered rigidly to its rules. Though she had been quite promiscuous, she accepted its proscription of all extramarital sex. One year later, feeling better than ever before, she entered once-a-week therapy. Her goal, which the therapist supported, was to maintain her accomplishments. The main obstacle to her doing this was her unconscious belief that by being successful and morally scrupulous, she was betraying her mother, her aunt, and also her childhood friends.

For example, even though she could afford it, she was unable to live outside a slum similar to one in which she had been raised. Also, as Talia began to rely on the therapist, she developed a constricting sense of disloyalty to her aunt and mother. On one occasion, after a particularly good session, she dreamed of the death of her aunt when she was 10.

Six months after beginning therapy, the patient's sense of pride in her chastity was threatened by a powerful, almost irrepressible urge to have sexual relations with a certain member of her church. The therapist, who was not aware that Talia had developed the sexual urge out of loyalty to her mother, erred by telling the patient that if she truly loved her friend she might consider having an affair with him. Talia became upset, and her sexual interest in her friend became more intense and tormenting. The therapist, who then realized her mistake, reminded Talia of her religious scruples and supported her in her goal of maintaining her good standing in her new family, the church. Talia rapidly improved. She became more aware that she was irrationally guilty about being morally superior to her mother. The therapist told the patient that she had been tempted to violate her scruples so as to lower herself to her mother's level. The patient understood this interpretation, and over a period of time used it to acquire control over her conscience. This enabled her to have sexual feelings toward her male friend without feeling that she had to have intercourse with him.

The next patient to be discussed, Mrs. C., also suffered from survivor guilt and an intense sense of responsibility for her parents and siblings. She felt that by being superior to them she was hurting them, and she developed penis envy in an attempt to restore them. (For a detailed discussion of Mrs. C., a patient studied by our research group, see Weiss, Sampson, & the Mount Zion Psychotherapy Research Group, 1986, especially Chapter 10.)

Mrs. C.

Mrs. C. was the third of four children born to an upper-middle-class family. She acquired a powerful sense of responsibility early in life, first for her helpless mother, then for her father and siblings.

Mrs. C. considered both parents pathetic, unable to enjoy life, and unendowed with a reasonable sense of authority. Her mother was unable to exert any control over her children; they pummeled each other in her presence as she stood by helplessly. Her father, when provoked by the children, was prone to violence. On one occasion when Mrs. C. was 6, she hit her mother in the stomach. Her mother was unable to protect herself and wept in pain. When her father heard about the incident, he beat the patient and threw her into a closet. A few days later the patient beat up her younger brother.

Mrs. C. protected her parents' fragile sense of authority by belittling herself in various ways, including by developing penis envy. Mrs. C.'s penis envy was completely conscious from age 10. She began then to carry a stick between her legs, which she referred to as her penis. By her penis envy she attempted both to restore her brother, who was 6 years younger, and to demonstrate admiration for her father. She also attempted by her penis envy to restore her mother. She unconsciously believed that her mother was upset by envy of her youth and attractiveness, and she punished herself for making her mother envious by envying her younger brother in much the same way as she assumed her mother envied her.

The next example illustrates that a patient may struggle to change a maladaptive pathogenic belief about reality by developing an attitude opposite to the one supported by the belief. In this example, a patient developed a sense of entitlement in an effort to change her belief that she was undeserving.

Marla L.

Marla L. was born to poor parents, both of whom worked hard in a small family business to make a marginal living. Her parents survived a serious financial crisis before Marla was born, and as a consequence became exceedingly frugal. They saved as much money as possible in order to be prepared for another crisis. In childhood and early adolescence, Marla was even more frugal than her parents. When she spent money on herself she would feel disloyal to her parents, and in addition would fear that she was robbing the family emergency fund.

In her adult life, Marla became a successful lawyer and married a wealthy businessman. She now could afford to spend money more freely, but was still constrained by survivor guilt about her spending while her parents continued to practice a rigid frugality.

After enduring her own frugality for several years, Marla began to work unconsciously at overcoming it by changing the beliefs underlying it. She used the direct approach of behaving in a way opposite to that prescribed by the beliefs: She became extravagant. She spent thousands of dollars on a gold necklace for herself, and on her second wedding anniversary she gave a very large and expensive party for herself and her husband.

Marla's extravagance persisted for 18 months. By then she had achieved her goal of demonstrating to herself that she did not have to be constrained by the beliefs she had acquired in childhood. Moreover, Marla derived some permanent gains from her experience. After her excessive spending, she did not return to her old frugal ways; rather, she came to exercise a reasonable and moderate control over her finances.

Marla's struggle to change the beliefs underlying her rigid frugality throws light on the issue of entitlement. During her period of extravagance, when questioned by her husband about the wisdom of her expenditures, Marla would self-righteously assert her right to spend her money as she pleased. Clearly, Marla's manifest sense of entitlement was not primary, but compensatory for the unconscious belief that she was not entitled. A patient who manifests a rigid and persistent sense of entitlement often is motivated much as Marla was. Such a patient almost invariably derives his sense of entitlement, not from having been overindulged (though overindulgence may have contributed to it), but as part of an effort to compensate for, counter, or change an unconscious belief that denies him indulgence.

A person's manifest behavior may express adaptive efforts to compensate for certain weaknesses that he maintains in compliance with his unconscious pathogenic beliefs. This may be illustrated by the case of Randall D., who came to analysis with a severe obsessive compulsive character disorder.

Randall D.

Randall's primary problem was indecisiveness. He developed this difficulty in early childhood in relation to his parents, whom he perceived as lacking all authority. He felt unprotected by his parents; he was frightened that they could not say no to him. He felt omnipotent. He learned to protect himself from his omnipotence, and also to protect his parent' authority, by becoming unable to make decisions. He thereby kept himself handicapped. As soon as he would decide on a particular course of action, he would search unconsciously for a good reason to take a different and opposing course. Thus, this patient's obsessive compulsive disorder did not stem primarily from an unconscious ambivalence, but from an unconscious belief that if he were able to make decisions he would be too powerful for his parents—and, by extension, for others as well.

Throughout his childhood and adolescence, Randall was almost paralyzed by his indecisiveness. However, in his early 20s he learned to compensate for it by developing and adhering to certain rigid schedules and rules. For example, on weekdays he would always get up at 6:30, go to work at 7:35, come home at 4:30, eat dinner at 6:00, go to bed at 10:00, read for half an hour, and turn off his light at 10:30. He followed a different but equally rigid schedule on weekends. With his schedule, and with the other rules that he followed, he could avoid making decisions other than those involved in developing his rules and deciding to adhere to them. At the same time he could maintain a fairly good, albeit rigid, level of functioning.

A person who is weakened and hence endangered by his pathogenic beliefs may attempt to protect himself by two different and incompatible strategies: He may demonstrate intense ambivalence, and he may engage in what is sometimes referred to as "splitting." However, neither the ambivalence nor the splitting is primary. Both are secondary to the pathogenic beliefs and the contradictory methods of dealing with the weaknesses that stem from them.

Ruth Z.

Ruth Z., a 35-year-old housewife and mother of a 6-year-old girl, came to analysis because of difficulties with her husband. She was an only child who had been raised by a depressed, dominating, and demanding mother. For as long as Ruth could remember, her mother would accuse her of being selfish, mean, and the cause of her (the mother's) unhappiness. Her father, who was sullen and quiet, left the family when Ruth was 7.

Though Ruth consciously repudiated her mother's accusations, she unconsciously believed them. She unconsciously assumed responsibility for her mother's unhappiness. When her mother blamed her, Ruth could not defend herself; she would simply weep and feel miserable.

In her relations with her husband, Ruth had great difficulty dealing with marital quarrels. She was so endangered by unconscious guilt and remorse that she could not admit to being in the wrong. Moreover, in her desperation she would fend off guilt and remorse by contradictory means. On the one hand, she would attempt to placate her husband and induce him to be affectionate by tearfully protesting her innocence and by pleading for his understanding. On the other hand, she would attempt to put him in the wrong; she would be scornful and vituperative and would blame him for her unhappiness. Moreover, Ruth would sometimes attempt both strategies in the same dispute, shifting rapidly from one to the other.

Ruth's manifest ambivalence and splitting were secondary to the pathogenic beliefs underlying her sense of guilt. As Ruth was helped by her therapist to feel less vulnerable to her conscience, both her ambivalence and her apparent splitting waned. By the end of her treatment, Ruth was getting along fairly well with her husband.

THE RELATIONSHIP BETWEEN SHAME AND GUILT

A sense of shame plays a powerful part in the development and maintenance of psychopathology. Shame, like guilt, anxiety, and fear, stems from pathogenic beliefs that a person acquires in childhood from traumatic experiences with parents and siblings. A person may develop such beliefs by identifying with shameful parents or by complying with their putdowns.

A child may develop a sense of shame if he infers that his parents are suffering from shame. For example, a boy whose parents never talked about his brain-damaged younger brother inferred that his parents were ashamed of the brother; as a consequence, he developed a belief that he too should be ashamed. Another child, who considered his parents contemptible, inferred that as a child of these parents, he should be ashamed of himself. Still another child, whose older sister was loved while he was derided, developed the belief that he was worthless and shameful.

Since a child develops shame from compliance with his parents or from identification with them, he feels compelled to maintain his sense of shame in order to maintain his ties to his parents. Therefore, the patient who struggles successfully to overcome his sense of shame may feel guilty to his parents, or he may lose his sense of connection to them so that he becomes sad. This may be exemplified by a patient who perceived both parents as fragile and weak. They were anxious and insecure unless at home. The patient, by identifying with his parents, developed a great deal of social anxiety when away from home. He felt shy and ill at ease with people. He feared that if anyone would tease him or put him down, he would be unable to defend himself. As he succeeded in his therapy in overcoming his social anxiety, he developed considerable survivor guilt toward his parents. He felt sorry for them. He considered it unfair that he had enjoyed the benefits of a successful therapy, whereas his parents had not. When his guilt about his parents became too strong, he would ameliorate it by reviving his social anxiety. In this, as in other cases I have studied, the patient's shame was held in place by survivor guilt.

In another example, a patient maintained shameful behavior similar to that of her parents and siblings in order to maintain her ties to them. The members of her family related to one another through a kind of sadistic teasing. No one expressed love simply and directly. The patient, too, while ashamed of her inappropriate teasing behavior, continued the family tradition of insulting others. This patient was helped in therapy to stop her sadistic teasing and to become friendly. She became aware of how much progress she had made when she told her boyfriend simply and directly, "I love you." After she did this, she became sad. In her therapy, she realized that she now felt cut off from her parents. She was sorry for them because they had behaved so inappropriately. She was sorry for herself for having suffered from inappropriate behavior, and also for feeling disconnected from them. She felt as if she were "cut off, floating in outer space."

SUMMARY

A person is powerfully motivated to adapt to reality; beginning in infancy, he works throughout life to do this. As part of this work he attempts to acquire reliable beliefs about this reality, which includes himself, his interpersonal world, and the moral imperatives of his world. These beliefs, which may be in varying degrees unconscious, are central to his mental life. He perceives himself and others, and he develops and maintains his personality and his psychopathology, in accordance with them.

This thesis is not compatible with the theory of the mind that Freud presented in his early writings (1900–1915), but is compatible with certain of Freud's late formulations (e.g., 1926a, 1940a) and with those of Hartmann (1939, 1956a, 1956b) and others. The difference between Freud's early theory and the views presented here may be illustrated by how each theory accounts for the urgency of maladaptive impulses. In Freud's early theory this urgency is derived from the close connection of impulse with instinct, and from the regulation of impulse by the pleasure principle. The theory presented here, while not denying the importance of instinct, assumes that this urgency is invariably supported by certain conscious and unconscious beliefs about reality and morality that are endowed with awesome authority.

Shame is of great importance in the development and maintenance of much psychopathology. However, it is almost always held in place either by guilt or by the wish to maintain ties to parents.

CHAPTER 3

The Therapist's Task

According to the present theory, the therapist's basic task is to help the patient in his working to disprove his pathogenic beliefs and to pursue the goals forbidden by these beliefs. Thus, in contrast to the traditional theory, the present theory assumes that the patient and therapist have the same purpose—namely, the disconfirmation by the patient of his pathogenic beliefs. Indeed, the disconfirmation of these beliefs is so important that the therapist may judge a particular technique by this simple criterion: Does it contribute directly or indirectly to the patient's disproving his pathogenic beliefs?

When the patient perceives the therapist as sympathetic to his plans, the patient almost invariably reacts immediately by feeling less anxious, more secure, and more confident in the therapist. The fact that the patient reacts this way immediately after a passed test or a pro-plan interpretation has been demonstrated by formal quantitative research (see Chapter 8). The patient may reveal his greater sense of security with the therapist directly, by being bolder, more insightful, and more confident with the therapist. Or, after a brief pause, he may reveal it by testing the therapist more vigorously. In cases where the patient perceives the therapist as opposed to his plans, he becomes less secure and more anxious and defensive, and is impeded in his efforts to test his pathogenic beliefs.

The therapist's approach is case-specific; that is, the therapist should help the patient to feel secure enough to face whatever dangers are foretold by his particular pathogenic beliefs, and to pursue whatever goals his particular beliefs have prevented him from pursuing effectively. The value of a case-specific approach may be illustrated by the following account of the first 4 years of the analysis of Roberta P.

Roberta P.

Roberta P., an unmarried lawyer in her early 30s, was the only child in a middle-class family. Her childhood was bleak. Both parents were withdrawn, unavailable, and burdened by the responsibility of raising her. In her analysis Roberta was cautious and distant, but doggedly cheerful in her attempts to interest the analyst.

Roberta's central pathogenic beliefs concerned the danger of rejection. She unconsciously believed that she was burdensome and that she would be and should be rejected. The analyst decided that to help Roberta to face this belief so that she could test it and ultimately change it, he should be friendly and accepting, and should avoid saying or doing anything that Roberta might experience as rejecting.

During the first 3 years of her analysis, Roberta made slow progress. She tested the analyst cautiously by requesting numerous schedule changes and by providing him with opportunities to humiliate her. The analyst readily accommodated Roberta's requests and avoided agreeing with her self-putdowns. As a consequence, Roberta became more open, friendlier to the analyst, and more aware that she had felt lonely and uncared for throughout her childhood.

In the fourth year of her analysis, Roberta offered the analyst a major rejection test. She announced that she had achieved her goals for therapy and that she planned to stop treatment in 3 months. The analyst implicitly opposed Roberta's stopping. He offered her a number of interpretations that connected her planning to stop with her fear of rejection. He told her that she feared she was a burden on him, that she wanted to reject him before he rejected her, and that she believed she did not deserve more help. Roberta showed interest in these interpretations but was not swayed by them. However, she acknowledged that she did not know why she wanted to stop. The analyst urged her to continue until her motives for stopping became clear. Roberta persisted in her plan to stop until just before her deadline, when she grudgingly agreed to continue for a while.

The therapist's urging Roberta to continue treatment reassured her that he would not reject her. Like the moviegoer who wept at the happy ending to the movie romance, Roberta became relieved and so able to tolerate previously repressed sadness. She brought forth a memory of maternal rejection. On one occasion when she was 6 years old, gang warfare erupted in her neighborhood. Everyone was frightened, and the other mothers made their children stay inside. However, Roberta's mother gave her money and sent her out to buy groceries. Roberta assumed that her mother wanted her to be killed. When she reported this episode, Roberta felt sad and wept.

During the next phase of her therapy, Roberta felt closer to the analyst. She remembered more episodes of parental rejection, and she accepted the interpretation that she had complied with her parents' lack of interest in her by believing herself unimportant and undeserving. She remembered an occasion in childhood when she had felt puzzled that a neighbor went out of her way to chat with her, and reported that she still felt surprised when someone was friendly.

According to the present theory, Roberta was helped by the analyst's interpretations, by his passing her tests, and by his overall friendly approach. The interpretations focused Roberta's attention on her belief that she would be rejected. However, she was not able to face this belief affectively or to remember its origins in her childhood traumas until the analyst passed a difficult rejection test. His doing so helped the patient feel secure enough with him to face the horrifying memory of her mother's endangering her life.

Freud's 1911–1915 theory contrasts with the present theory in its assessment of the techniques described above. According to the 1911–1915 theory, the analyst's friendliness would be a manipulation that might gratify Roberta's unconscious dependency, thereby either preventing her from facing her dependency, or depriving her of motivation for working in treatment. In addition, the 1911–1915 theory would view Roberta's frequent requests for schedule changes and her threats to quit treatment as resistances that should be interpreted. According to this theory, such behavior might express Roberta's unconscious hostility to the analyst, or it might protect her against her unconscious dependency on him, or both. Also, according to the 1911–1915 theory, the analyst's acceptance at face value of Roberta's account of parental rejection would be viewed as permitting her to blame her parents for her problems (i.e., to externalize the problems) and so to avoid facing her part in them. For example, it might be viewed as preventing her from discovering that she had been demanding with her parents and rejecting of them, and that she therefore had provoked their rejection.

A COMPARISON OF THE 1911–1915 THEORY AND THE THEORY PROPOSED HERE: NEUTRALITY VERSUS SIDING WITH THE PATIENT'S PLAN

Freud's 1911–1915 theory recommends that the therapist be neutral[1] when analyzing an unconscious conflict. According to this theory, such conflict generally occurs between powerful instinctual impulses that seek conflicting gratifications. Since in the 1911–1915 theory unconscious impulses are not organized by purpose or plan, no one impulse is necessarily more pertinent to the patient's goals than another; therefore, the therapist has no reason to favor one impulse over another. In fact, he has good reason not to take sides: He is strongly opposed to imposing his own views on the patient. He assumes that by making the patient aware of both sides of the conflict, he

---

[1]The 1911–1915 theory's recommendation of neutrality toward unconscious conflict reflects Freud's intention to develop a rational approach, respectful of the patient's autonomy. Freud was critical of the methods of certain contemporary psychotherapists who tried to influence their patients by use of authority, reassurance, or mystifying ritual, or who imposed their own values or ideas on their patients. He considered such techniques manipulative and likely to strengthen a patient's defenses. He assumed, too, that rather than helping the patient become stronger and more independent, such techniques tend to keep the patient dependent. To avoid doing this, Freud recommended that the therapist rely mainly on interpretation; that he avoid the use of reassurance or authority; and that he remain relatively detached, neutral, and objective.

provides the patient with the tools to resolve his conflict through conscious thought.

In contrast, the present theory conceptualizes unconscious conflict as typically occurring between certain of the patient's normal, desirable goals and his expectation that by pursuing these goals he will put himself or someone he loves in danger. In this conflict the therapist is on the side of the patient's goals, and his primary task is to help the patient pursue his goals by enabling him to realize that the dangers foretold by his pathogenic beliefs are not real.

The 1911–1915 theory's recommendation of neutrality or impartiality is reflected in its assumption that the therapist should analyze from the surface, taking up each new resistance as it manifests itself. Just as the therapist has no reason to take sides in an unconscious conflict, he has no reason to focus more on some unconscious resistances than on others.

In contrast, the present theory perceives the surface not as manifesting unconscious resistances, but as reflecting tests of pathogenic beliefs. Just how the therapist reacts to a test depends on his understanding of the patient's beliefs and also of the tests that the patient is giving him. In some instances the therapist may pass a test by agreeing with the patient's ideas about himself and even by elaborating on them. However, in other instances the therapist may pass a test by challenging the patient's formulations—for example, when the patient presents a problem in compliance to a parent's or a spouse's false ideas about him—as in the case of Willa A.

Willa A.

Willa A. wished unconsciously to leave an obviously inadequate, ungiving, and dependent husband, and was helped by her therapy to do so. Willa entered treatment burdened unconsciously by an exaggerated sense of responsibility for her husband. However, she did not know consciously why she was unhappy in her marriage. She could not decide whether, as her mother had often told her, she was too selfish to get along with anyone, or whether her husband was in fact difficult.

The patient, who was struggling to see her husband clearly, tested the therapist in various ways. Sometimes she implied quite reasonably that her husband was at fault. The therapist would pass this test by accepting the patient's account. At other times she accepted responsibility for problems for which in fact she was not responsible, as, for example, when she complained that she was unresponsive in sex with her husband. The therapist passed this test by not taking Willa's account at face value. Instead, by questioning her he demonstrated that her husband had little or no sexual interest in her, and that she had been responsive to his occasional advances.

The Use of Reassurance or Authority

As already noted, the 1911–1915 theory recommends that the therapist avoid the use of reassurance or authority. For example, he should generally neither make recommendations nor offer prohibitions. Rather, he should rely mainly on interpretation to accomplish his essential task of making the unconscious conscious.

In contrast, the theory proposed here assumes that the therapist should employ a variety of means besides interpretation, including in some instances reassurance or the use of authority. Consider, for example, the analysis presented above of Roberta P., who suffered from the pathogenic belief that she would be and should be rejected by the analyst. Though the analyst interpreted this belief, Roberta did not acquire insight into it until the analyst used his authority to pass a serious rejection test, urging Roberta to continue her analysis. After this, Roberta began to experience the validity of the analyst's previous interpretations. She then felt safe enough to remember how rejected she had been by her mother, and to realize that she had avoided feeling friendly toward the analyst for fear he would reject her.

Though the use of authority or reassurance is pro-plan in some instances, it is anti-plan in others. For example, some patients experience reassurance as patronizing, and some patients consider the use of authority as infantilizing or humiliating. Just how the therapist may help the patient feel safe depends on how the patient felt endangered in his childhood. For example, a patient who had felt rejected by austere, formal parents was helped to feel safe by the therapist's chatting with him about topics of mutual interest. Another patient who had suffered from demanding parents whom he could not please was helped by the therapist's appreciating the patient's efforts to please him.

Some patients, especially those who were unable in childhood to develop a reliable sense of connection with their parents, assume that they do not deserve to feel connected to another person. They assume that they will be rejected by the therapist. Such a patient may not feel secure enough with the therapist to receive help unless the therapist makes unusual efforts to enable the patient to feel connected to him. For example, one patient who in early childhood could not form a connection to his irritable, self-centered parents was quite anxious and restless, and he was unable to find a job that he liked. He was helped somewhat by psychotherapy and by attending support groups. However, the patient did not obtain a good job until his therapist suggested that the patient phone him every day and give a 10-minute report on his activities. After doing this for several months, the patient became less depressed and succeeded in finding a job that he liked.

A patient who in childhood infers from parental neglect that he does not deserve protection may feel unsafe in therapy until the therapist uses his authority to demonstrate that he will protect the patient. This was the case with Geoffrey B., described below.

Geoffrey B.

Geoffrey B., a young physician and a father of two, became self-destructively promiscuous shortly after beginning an analysis. He began to have so many affairs and to be so indiscreet that he was acquiring a reputation that threatened his marriage and his career. However, he blandly implied to the analyst that his promiscuity was not a problem.

The analyst assumed that the patient was testing him to determine whether the analyst would protect him. He confronted the patient repeatedly with his self-destructiveness. However, the patient provocatively continued to be promiscuous. Finally the analyst told Geoffrey that unless he stopped his promiscuity, he (the analyst) would discontinue the treatment. The patient became angry, wept, and berated the analyst for his failure to maintain an "analytic" attitude. However, rather than stopping treatment, he stopped being promiscuous. Also, he became more secure and more trusting in the analysis, and he retrieved several childhood memories of his parents' failure to protect him from self-destructive sexual behavior. He remembered that in the fourth grade he would expose himself in the school corridors. His teachers tried to enlist his parents' help in dealing with this, but his parents did not respond.

After the episode described above, Geoffrey settled down in treatment and continued by other means to work at disconfirming the belief that he did not deserve help or protection.

The therapist's use of authority in the treatments of Geoffrey B. and of Roberta P. helped them to feel safe. Both Geoffrey and Roberta did well. Patients who require reassurance or the use of authority are not necessarily more disturbed than patients who do not. The fact that the patient is not suitable for treatment by the traditional technique may reflect the limitations of that technique rather than the patient's degree of disturbance.

The present theory also weakens the distinction between uncovering therapy and supportive therapy. This distinction makes sense in the 1911–1915 theory, with its assumption that a patient may become conscious of the repressed only by use of interpretation. However, it does not make sense in the present theory, which assumes that in some instances the patient may feel safe enough with the therapist to lift his repressions without benefit of interpretation, and thus to get insights on his own. This assumption is compatible with Wallerstein's (1986) finding that patients who received so-called supportive therapy demonstrated as much structural change in follow-up interviews as did patients who received uncovering therapy.

In some instances the patient benefits primarily from the good relationship he establishes with the therapist and the new experiences he acquires in this relationship. He may then develop insights secondarily by re-evaluating his present and past situations in the light of his new experiences. Consider, for example, a patient who inferred from his relations with his rejecting parents that he deserved to be rejected. As he came to experience the therapist as accepting him, he began to change this pathogenic belief and to feel more self-esteem. He also re-evaluated his childhood. He began to question his parents' treatment of him and to realize that he had deserved better (see Alexander & French, 1946, p. 20).

The Use of Authority versus Protecting the Patient's Autonomy

In its concern for protecting the patient's autonomy, the 1911–1915 theory may induce the therapist to take the patient's conscious wishes too literally. A patient may test the therapist by presenting plans contrary to his unconscious goals. For example, a patient who unconsciously wishes to test the belief that he will be rejected may threaten to decrease the frequency of his visits, hoping unconsciously that the therapist will dissuade him from doing this. If the therapist takes the patient's conscious wishes at face value, he may permit the patient to do something he (the patient) does not want to do. This was the case in the treatment of Timothy E., whose analyst, out of respect for his autonomy, went along with his conscious wish to marry an obviously unsatisfactory woman.

Timothy E.

Timothy E., an unmarried male in his late 20s, had suffered in childhood at the hands of a mother who was depressed, vituperative, and insulting. He had developed the beliefs that he was responsible for his mother and that he had failed to make her happy, and so deserved her rejection. The patient had unconsciously hoped that his father, who was withdrawn, would intervene with his mother on his behalf. However, his father did not intervene, and thus failed to protect the patient from his belief that unless he made his mother happy he deserved to be rejected by her.

In his analysis, Timothy E. developed sufficient confidence in the male analyst to test these beliefs by dating an obviously unsatisfactory woman who, like his mother, was abusive and ungiving.

The patient hoped that the therapist would intervene by pointing out that he was not responsible for the happiness of his girlfriend, who was almost impossible to get along with. However, the therapist did not intervene, and the patient felt compelled to marry the woman. Timothy did not become completely conscious of all this until several years after his marriage, when his wife left him for another man. He then started to date a cheerful and giving woman, and was deeply impressed by the contrast between his wife and his new girlfriend. He became aware that he had found his wife almost intolerable, and that he had hoped and expected that the therapist would warn him against marrying her. In the treatment of Timothy E., the therapist, who out of respect for the patient's autonomy took his conscious statements at face value, had in fact failed to protect his autonomy.

The same point may be illustrated by the analysis of Roberta P. If her analyst had taken literally her wish to stop treatment, and had not tried to get her to continue, she would have felt betrayed and unable to disprove the disturbing unconscious belief that she did not deserve to receive help. By the same token, Willa A. (the woman who wished to leave an unsatisfactory husband) would have been harmed if the therapist had taken her professions of love for her husband at face value, or if the therapist had agreed that she had been provoking her husband's unsatisfactory behavior. Similarly, Geoffrey B. (the man whose promiscuity threatened his reputation) would have been harmed if his therapist had not insisted that he stop being promiscuous. He would unconsciously have felt betrayed, and his pathogenic belief that he did not deserve to be protected would have been confirmed.

A better guide to the patient's goals than his conscious statements is his reactions to the therapist's interventions. Roberta P. was relieved when her analyst urged her to continue treatment, and soon after retrieved an important new memory, which threw light on her psychopathology. Willa A. felt better when her therapist did not agree with her that she was responsible for her marital difficulties, and she then became more insightful. Geoffrey B. settled down when his analyst insisted he stop his promiscuous behavior, and he then retrieved an important memory of childhood neglect.

The Importance of Helping the Patient to Realize that He Developed His Psychopathology in His Relations with His Parents

Closely related to the 1911–1915 theory's recommendation that the therapist protect the patient's autonomy is its recommendation that the therapist encourage the patient to take responsibility for his problems. The two ideas are related, because the patient cannot be independent unless he takes such responsibility. However, just as the therapist guided by the 1911–1915 theory may be too literal in his attempts to protect the patient's autonomy, he may be too literal in his attempts to uphold the ideal of patient responsibility. For example, the therapist may be concerned that if the patient is permitted to blame his parents for his problems, he will externalize the problems and so escape responsibility both for his problems and for working to solve them.

According to the present theory, the patient who explores the traumas of his childhood does so not to escape responsibility for his problems, but as part of his working to understand these problems and to solve them. He takes a step forward when he begins to realize that he suffered from parental mistreatment, complied with it, and as a consequence developed the pathogenic belief that he deserves mistreatment. His realization that he suffers from pathogenic beliefs inferred from traumatic experiences with his parents helps him to take responsibility for solving his problems. He also learns how he may solve them—that is, by changing these beliefs.

However, if the therapist discourages the patient from recognizing the part his parents played in the development of his psychopathology, the patient may be impeded in his effort to solve his problems. He may continue to believe, as he did in early childhood, that he deserved the parental treatment he received. Suppose, for example, that Roberta P. had been told by her therapist that she had provoked her parents to reject her, either by rejecting them or by being hostile to them; or suppose that she had been told that she was focusing on her parents' neglect of her so as to avoid facing her own neglect of them. If she had taken such comments to heart, she would have been impeded in her efforts to disprove the belief that she deserved to be rejected.

Resistance Analysis

According to the 1911–1915 theory, the therapist, in carrying out the task of making the unconscious conscious, relies heavily on the interpretation of the patient's resistances. From the perspective of the theory proposed here, such resistance interpretations may be counterproductive, especially in the treatment of patients who experience resistance interpretations as criticisms. Such interpretations may prevent the patient from feeling safe enough with the therapist to discuss his feelings of being inadequate, guilty, or unappreciated. This was the case in the analysis of Lowell A.

Lowell A.

Lowell A. was an energetic, imaginative, and intelligent sociologist whose problems arose from compliance with a highly critical father. The patient came to his first analysis complaining of social inhibition, shyness, fear of rejection by women, and anxiety about working. His first analyst, who was much less critical than the patient's father, provided the patient with enough security to receive help in all of these areas. Lowell got married, had several children, and became a tenured professor. When Lowell sought a second analysis 15 years after completion of the first, he spoke well of his first analyst, a respected teacher in the local psychoanalytic institute.

Lowell sought additional treatment because he was at times moderately depressed, unduly diffident with his students and colleagues, and unable to enjoy life as much as he thought he should. In the opening phase of the second analysis, Lowell tested the analyst by presenting him with numerous opportunities to put him down. When the analyst did not do so, Lowell relaxed, became more expansive, and gained more confidence in the analyst. He then began to criticize the first analyst for not encouraging him in his own attempts to understand himself. He complained that the first analyst had always viewed his (Lowell's) explanations for his problems as inadequate—that is, as consisting of half-truths, rationalizations, or denials. At one point Lowell stated with considerable feeling, "I'm an intelligent person. I've always thought about my problems. I enjoy problem solving, and I like to work with friends to solve problems. I usually have lots of ideas. However, my analyst had to do all the work. I had none of the fun of discovering, of thinking, of problem solving. Nothing I said was ever quite right, even if I said something my analyst had already told me."

The second analyst encouraged Lowell to present his own ideas, which were generally interesting and pertinent. The patient became progressively more friendly and secure with the analyst. He remembered more about his father's criticizing him. His father was never satisfied with him. He criticized the gifts the patient gave him, his clothes, his complexion, his interests, his friends, his being overweight, and even his taste in movies and music. The patient had remembered his father's "picking on him" but had not remembered that he had been affected by it. Now he realized that he had felt humiliated, sad, and angry.

Lowell also came to realize that he had developed an irrational and persistent expectation of criticism. He became more relaxed and friendly with his colleagues, his students, and his wife and children. He began to enjoy taking his two sons to baseball games and picnics, and they rewarded him by becoming more affectionate. Lowell's depressions subsided, and he enjoyed life more.

The techniques employed by Lowell's first analyst were in keeping with the 1911–1915 theory. His considerable use of interpretation was based on two assumptions: first, that the patient's productions were compromise formations, and thus inevitably incomplete; and second, that the patient could not lift his repressions himself. Therefore, the patient could not become aware of the contents he had repressed unless the analyst interpreted them. The analyst's cool, detached attitude was based on his assumption that if he were friendly, he would be gratifying the patient's dependency and thus would deprive the patient of his motivation to work in therapy. He assumed that the patient would do best when he was experiencing an optimal level of anxiety; too much anxiety would increase his resistance, and too little anxiety would weaken his motivation.

The second analyst's technique reflects the assumptions of the theory proposed here—that the more the analyst is able to help a patient to realize that the dangers predicted by his pathogenic beliefs are not real, the more the patient will be able to face these dangers, and the more he will be able to work at disconfirming his pathogenic beliefs by testing them. A patient does not need to be goaded to work in treatment. He is intensely interested in solving his problems, and if helped to feel secure he may work successfully to solve them largely on his own. When left to himself, he will set his own agenda.

When Lowell was offered the opportunity in his second analysis to set his agenda, he did so. He unconsciously set out to assure himself by testing the analyst that the analyst would not put him down. As the patient began to feel safer with the analyst, he became friendlier, and the analyst returned his friendliness. This helped the patient to feel secure enough to remember and describe his humiliating experiences with his father. As Lowell succeeded in tracing the development of his pathogenic beliefs to certain experiences with his father, he became less bound by these beliefs and friendlier to his colleagues, students, and family. His aloofness toward his sons had reflected the belief that his father had treated him the way sons should be treated. As he changed this belief, he began to enjoy his sons more. Also, his chronic depression reflected the belief that he was unable to do things right; as he disconfirmed this belief, he became more cheerful and optimistic.

Explanations in Terms of Impulse and Defense

Whereas in the 1911–1915 theory explanations in terms of impulse and defense (or of a compromise between these) are fundamental, this is not the case in the theory proposed here. From the perspective of the present theory, explanations in terms of impulse, defense, and compromise, though sometimes helpful, are often unsatisfying. The patient is left with the question of why certain impulses or defenses are especially important in his mental life. For example, he may wonder, "Why am I especially hostile?" or "Why am I especially dependent?" or "Why have I become withdrawn?" Moreover, the patient may feel put down by explanations in terms of impulse and defense—hostility, dependency, and withdrawal are not highly regarded—so that he becomes insecure with the therapist.

In most cases the patient is more satisfied with explanations that assume his behavior was acquired from certain childhood experiences, and that it serves an adaptive function or an unconscious moral purpose. Such explanations, according to the present theory, are more accurate, make more intuitive sense to the patient, and are more helpful. For example, a particular patient may learn more and also feel safer if he is told not simply, "You are very hostile toward your wife," but "You are ruining your marriage by fighting with your wife. You are being loyal to your father, who ruined his marriage by such fighting." Similarly, a certain patient may learn more and feel safer if he is told not simply, "You are very dependent," but "You are overly dependent because you believe others want you to need them." A third patient may learn more if he is told not simply, "You are withdrawn," but "You are withdrawn because you were unable to interest your self-centered parents, and you concluded that you weren't supposed to try to interest them."

An example of a resistance interpretation that may be counterproductive is the interpretation, sometimes offered to a patient who talks over his problems with a friend, that he is "splitting the transference." A patient who tells the therapist about confiding in a friend may be testing his right to be separate from the therapist; if so, he may be set back by this interpretation. He may infer that he is hurting the therapist, and so he may experience his pathogenic belief as confirmed. He may then develop more irrational guilt about separating from the therapist.

The Value of a Case-Specific Approach

As noted above, a theory of technique that prescribes roughly the same approach (or a range of related approaches) for every patient is not sufficiently flexible. It may be well suited to the treatment of some patients, but not to the treatment of others.

Thus the techniques prescribed by the 1911–1915 theory are not well suited to the treatment of patients who require reassurance, strong acceptance, or the use of authority. They are not well suited to the therapy of patients who have complied with their parents' mistreatment and who may overcome their compliance only by coming to understand how their parents mistreated them. Nor are they well suited to the therapy of patients who may overcome their self-destructiveness only if the therapist focuses on their unconscious feelings of guilt and their need to sacrifice their interests to those of others.

Despite its weaknesses, the 1911–1915 theory, with its recommendations that the therapist be detached, impersonal, non-critical, and consistent, is useful (if not optimal) in the treatment of a variety of patients. The consistency prescribed by the 1911–1915 theory may enable the patient to develop a plan for testing his pathogenic beliefs that is adapted to the therapist's approach, style, and personality. The patient may be enabled by the therapist's consistency to anticipate just how the therapist will respond to his initiatives, and thus to develop tests that the therapist is likely to pass. If the patient, by testing the therapist, comes to delineate unconsciously the therapist's weaknesses and strengths, the patient may devise tests that utilize the therapist's strengths and avoid his weaknesses.

These points are illustrated by the treatment of Karen B., who discovered unconsciously that her analyst was especially likely to pass a particular kind of test, and so came to rely more and more on that kind of test.

Karen B.

Karen, a married woman in her early 30s, came to analysis burdened by the pathogenic belief that she was omnipotently responsible for the happiness and well-being of her parents, siblings, and husband, all of whom she perceived as fragile and easily hurt. In order to protect them, she made herself weak, indecisive, and jealous. In her analysis, Karen tested her belief in her omnipotence in several different ways. First, she would tell the analyst about episodes in which she took a strong position with her husband, either in their sex life or in their social life. Karen hoped that the analyst would approve of her being strong with her husband. However, he did not; rather, he interpreted her behavior as reflecting her penis envy, and thus as stemming from her sense of inadequacy. Karen inferred from this that the analyst did not want her to be strong with her husband.

Karen also tested her omnipotence by offering the analyst passive-into-active tests. In these, Karen acted hurt by the analyst as, in her opinion, her parents had been hurt by her. For example, she complained in a weepy voice that the analyst was unfairly charging her for a missed appointment. In such tests, Karen was attempting to determine whether her analyst felt omnipotently responsible for her as she had felt for her parents. She hoped that he did not; if he did not, Karen could identify with him, and so take less seriously her (internalized) parents' complaints about her. The analyst almost always passed this kind of test: In the face of Karen's complaints about him, he was unmoved and unapologetic. Karen was helped by this. In the sessions immediately following the therapist's passing this kind of test, the patient would be more cheerful, would feel stronger, and in some instances would demonstrate greater insight into her exaggerated sense of responsibility for others.

Karen unconsciously came to realize that her analyst consistently passed her passive-into-active tests, but not those tests in which she bragged about dominating her husband. Therefore, she became increasingly reliant on the former kind of test. Moreover, whenever the analyst began to lose his focus, Karen would get him back on course by carrying out a passive-into-active test. In her work with her analyst, Karen used her analyst's particular strengths to good effect. Though her analyst did not interpret Karen's belief in her omnipotence, he helped her, by passing her passive-into-active tests, to become conscious of this belief and to make progress in disconfirming it.

Among the variety of patients who may benefit from the 1911–1915 approach is the patient who suffers from the pathogenic belief that if he challenges or insults the therapist he will be punished. The therapist who subscribes to the 1911–1915 theory is likely to pass such tests by remaining detached and noncritical in the face of the patient's challenges. This therapist is also likely to be helpful to a patient who suffers unconsciously from the belief that he has no right to protect himself from the intrusions of others, and who tests the therapist by tempting him to be intrusive. He is likely to be helpful, too, with a patient who suffers from the belief that he will seduce the therapist, and who tests this belief by being seductive; or with the patient who fears he will worry the therapist, and who tests this belief by being worrisome.

KOHUT'S RECOMMENDATIONS

Just as the traditional theory is well suited to the treatment of some kinds of patients but not others, so are Kohut's recommendations (Kohut, 1959, 1971, 1984). These were first applied to the treatment of patients with narcissistic disorders, and later extended to the treatment of a variety of patients. From the perspective of the present theory, Kohut's ideas mark an advance in both theory and technique over the 1911–1915 theory. Kohut emphasizes more than did the 1911–1915 theory that psychopathology may arise from the child's disturbed relations to his parents. Also in contrast to the 1911–1915 theory, Kohut points to the curative nature of the patient's experiences with the therapist (Kohut, 1984). Moreover, Kohut's method is helpful with certain kinds of patients for whom the 1911–1915 theory is not well suited. These include patients who were especially rejected in childhood and who need to feel especially accepted by the therapist. It also includes patients who suffered in childhood from being ashamed of their parents and who need to idealize the therapist.

Kohut's recommendations center around the handling of what he calls certain "transference or transference-like phenomena," or, more specifically, "the idealizing transference" and the "mirror transference" (Kohut, 1971). The patient who develops a mirror transference needs to be listened to and admired by the therapist; the patient who develops an idealizing transference needs to idealize the therapist. In each instance, the therapist, according to Kohut (1984), should accept the role the patient assigns him. In the case of the idealizing transference, the therapist should permit the idealization. In the case of the mirror transference, the therapist should accept the patient's egocentricity, pride, and exhibitionism. If the patient is reluctant to express pride, the therapist may encourage him to do so by tactfully accepting his exhibitionistic grandiosity or by interpreting his resistances to the revelation of his grandiosity

The analyst guided by the 1911–1915 theory might criticize Kohut's recommendation for dealing with the idealizing transference, on the grounds that it does not take account of the patient's underlying hostility. Also, he might criticize Kohut's recommendation for dealing with the mirror transference, on the grounds that it gratifies the patient's dependency and exhibitionism. In contrast, the present theory assumes that certain patients may develop a mirror transference in order to test the pathogenic belief that they do not deserve to be listened to, taken seriously, or respected. If, as Kohut recommends, the therapist listens to such a patient, takes him seriously, and encourages him to experience pride, he may help the patient feel more secure with him. The therapist may thereby help the patient feel safe enough to test his pathogenic beliefs and move toward changing them.

A patient may develop an idealizing transference to test the belief that he does not deserve a relationship with a decent, admirable authority. He may develop this belief in childhood if he perceives his parents as ashamed, weak, foolish, or seriously flawed. To the child, such parents may be highly traumatic. His parents are such an important part of his life that his security and self-esteem depend on his being able to rely on them and admire them. Unless he can perceive them as strong, wise, and self-respecting, he may find it difficult to respect himself. By idealizing the therapist, he may make progress in overcoming his sense of shame and in becoming aware that he was ashamed of his parents.

However, Kohut's recommendations may be of little or no value when applied to patients who, though manifestly similar to those described by Kohut, differ in their underlying pathologies. For example, a patient who suffers mainly from an exaggerated sense of responsibility for the happiness of others may attempt to discharge his responsibility to the therapist by admiring him. If the therapist then encourages this admiration, the patient may infer that the therapist needs it. The patient then may experience his pathogenic belief as confirmed, and so come to believe all the more in his responsibility for others.

Also, a patient who suffers from separation guilt may unconsciously deny his wish to separate by behaving as though he deeply needs the therapist's admiration and approval. The patient may be set back if the therapist takes the patient's neediness at face value and behaves in the nurturing way that the patient seems to require. The patient may infer that the therapist enjoys being nurturing, and so he may continue to be needy out of compliance.

Nor are Kohut's recommendations useful with patients who have suffered severe narcissistic wounds and who work at disconfirming the resulting pathogenic beliefs by giving passive-into-active tests. In such tests, the patient abuses the therapist as his parents abused him. He hopes that the therapist will not comply with his abuse as he complied with that of his parents. His purpose is to use the therapist's example to convince himself that such compliance is not mandatory, and thus that he need not comply with his (internalized) parents. If the therapist responds to passive-into-active tests by appearing too empathic with the patient's criticisms, he may seem to be taking these criticisms too seriously (or to be complying with them) and so may fail these tests.

Kohut's theory, in contrast to the present theory, characterizes psychopathology primarily in terms of deficits. The present theory, while assuming that long-standing pathogenic beliefs may result secondarily in the patient's failure to acquire certain psychological functions, characterizes psychopathology primarily in terms of pathogenic beliefs. This difference makes for a difference in the therapist's approach to the patient. The therapist who believes that the patient suffers from a deficit may assume that the patient requires favorable experiences with the therapist over a long period of time to make up for the deficit. The therapist who assumes that the patient suffers from a pathogenic belief assumes in some instances that the patient, by learning that he need not be guided by his pathogenic beliefs, may make quite rapid progress.

OTHER NON-CASE-SPECIFIC APPROACHES

Just as the 1911–1915 theory and Kohut's recommendations are insufficiently case-specific, any recommendations intended to apply to all patients or to all patients in a particular diagnostic category are insufficiently case-specific. Consider, for example, the recommendation of certain analysts (e.g., Langs, 1973, 1979) that the therapist take special care to maintain the frame of the therapy. A patient may benefit from this approach if in childhood his privacy was violated by an intrusive or sexually abusive parent, and if as a consequence he developed the belief that he should not protect himself from the intrusions of others. He may test this belief by tempting the therapist to weaken or ignore the framework of the therapy, and he will benefit from the therapist's not doing so. However, patients who suffer from the pathogenic belief that they will and should be rejected may benefit from a relatively loose frame. They may experience the imposition of a rigid frame as rejecting or withholding, and take it as evidence for their pathogenic beliefs.

Or consider Kernberg's recommendation (Kernberg, 1977, 1987) that the therapist should help a patient who has been diagnosed as borderline experience his repressed rage. This recommendation may be useful in the treatment of a patient who acquired his pathogenic beliefs by complying in childhood with parental abuse, and who works in therapy to become aware that he was abused, as part of his effort to stop complying with abuse. By expressing rage at his parents, he may become more aware that he was mistreated by them, and that he complied with the mistreatment.

The therapist's encouragement of the patient's rage may also be helpful in the treatment of a patient whose parents abused him by being enraged at him, and who tests the therapist by turning passive into active. This is because the patient is likely to infer that the therapist who comfortably tolerates or encourages his rage is not traumatized by it.

However, Kernberg's recommendation that the therapist encourage the patient's rage may not be helpful even in the treatment of a patient who complied in childhood with parental abuse, if that patient does not plan to work in therapy in one of the ways described above. For example, a patient who suffers from childhood compliance to abusive parents may plan to free himself from this compliance, not primarily by becoming enraged at his parents or at the therapist, but by trying to elicit the therapist's admiration and respect. The patient who wants to work in this way may be thrown off course if the therapist, instead of encouraging the patient's pride, encourages his anger.

THE CORRECTIVE EMOTIONAL EXPERIENCE

The theory proposed here agrees with Alexander and French (1946) that the therapist may help the patient by enabling him to obtain certain significant corrective emotional experiences. However, in contrast to the theory of Alexander and French, the present theory puts the value of the therapist's offering the patient certain corrective experiences in a broad theoretical context in which his offering the patient such experiences makes sense. It does not make sense in the context of the 1911–1915 theory. According to that theory, the unconscious mind does not contain beliefs that can be changed by corrective experiences. Rather, it contains psychic forces—namely, impulses and defenses that are regulated by the pleasure principle. According to the 1911–1915 theory, the therapist who attempts to offer the patient corrective experiences runs the risk of either strengthening the patient's defenses or satisfying his impulses, and thus of depriving the patient of motivation for therapy.

However, offering the patient corrective experiences does make sense in the context of the present theory, which assumes that the patient is working unconsciously to disprove certain unconscious pathogenic beliefs by seeking experiences that run counter to these beliefs. Our research supports the efficacy of such experiences (see Chapter 8). It demonstrates that the patient is profoundly affected by his perception of how the therapist responds to his tests. Regardless of how the therapist conceptualizes his approach, the patient unconsciously experiences the therapist's behavior as either passing his tests, failing his tests, or not pertaining to them. When the patient experiences the therapist as passing his tests, he makes immediate progress; when he experiences the therapist as failing them, he is immediately set back (see Chapter 8).

The present theory differs from Alexander and French's (1946) approach in that Alexander and French do not recognize the patient's unconscious testing of the therapist. Therefore, they do not recognize that the therapist should offer the patient the particular experiences that the patient is seeking by his testing. The present theory also differs from Alexander and French's in its assumption that the therapist may check on the pertinence of his interventions by observing the patient's reactions to them.

Critics of Alexander and French's formulation have argued that their technique requires the therapist to "role-play." This criticism applies neither to their approach nor to the ideas proposed here. The therapist who uses his theory and his empathy to understand the patient's unconscious motivations is not role-playing when he responds appropriately to the patient's tests. Consider, for example, the therapist who realizes that though his patient is threatening to quit, he is hoping unconsciously that the therapist will not let him do so. This therapist is not role-playing when he urges the patient to continue; rather, he is being appropriate and empathic. Indeed, to pass the patient's tests in accordance with the present theory requires no more role playing than to maintain the detached, impersonal attitude prescribed by the 1911–1915 theory in the face of a patient's dramatic and upsetting disclosures.

Nor does the therapist's approaching the patient in a way designed to pass one kind of test cast the patient–therapist relationship in a certain mold, so that the patient is less able to offer a new kind of test that requires a different approach. The patient can always find a way of changing his relationship to the therapist when his unconscious plan requires him to do so. This may be illustrated by the first year of the analysis of Teresa K.

Teresa K.

Teresa K.'s problems arose primarily from her childhood compliance with extremely demeaning parents. She would sometimes offer the therapist transference tests by manifesting her fear that the therapist would demean her. The therapist would pass this kind of test by demonstrating acceptance, and the patient would respond by feeling increased self-esteem, by becoming friendlier, and by bringing forth new memories of parental rejection.

However, the patient was never deterred by the therapist's friendliness from testing the therapist by becoming hostile and abusive. When it suited her purposes, she would demean the therapist as her parents had demeaned her. She would test the therapist in this way when she was contemplating a step forward that she assumed would show her (internalized) parents that she was not complying with their contempt. The therapist would pass this kind of test by standing up to Teresa's insults, thereby showing her that he was not complying with them. Teresa would identify with the therapist's noncompliance and would make the contemplated advance. Later she would again offer the therapist tests designed to induce him to demonstrate friendliness. The patient would sometimes go from one kind of test to the other and back again in a period of several weeks.

As illustrated above, the therapist's friendliness to Teresa, when she was friendly to him, did not deter her from being insulting and stubborn when this suited her purposes.

SUMMARY

According to the present theory, the therapist's basic task is to help the patient in his struggle to disprove his pathogenic beliefs and to pursue the goals forbidden by these beliefs. In carrying out this task, the therapist does a number of things: He helps the patient feel safe with him by demonstrating that he disagrees with the patient's pathogenic beliefs and sympathizes with his goals. He does these things not only by interpretation, but by his overall approach and attitude to the patient, and by passing the patient's tests. Also, he varies his approach from patient to patient: He adapts it to each patient's particular pathogenic beliefs, goals, and plans.

The 1911–1915 theory assumes that the therapist's basic task is to help the patient make the unconscious conscious. It assumes that the therapist may best accomplish this by being neutral to the patient's conflicts; by avoiding the use of authority or reassurance; and by relying primarily on interpretations, especially interpretations of the patient's resistances. From the perspective of the present theory, the 1911–1915 theory's recommendations may help some patients but not others. In some instances they may actually be harmful. Whether the 1911–1915 technique is helpful or not depends on the patient's particular pathogenic beliefs, plans, and goals.

In general the therapist should not be neutral, but should be the patient's ally in his efforts to disprove his pathogenic beliefs and to pursue his goals. Nor should the therapist avoid the use of reassurance or authority in situations where reassurance or authority may be helpful. Thus, interpretation is not the sine qua non of therapy. In some instances the patient may be helped to disconfirm his pathogenic beliefs and to pursue his goals primarily by his experiences with his therapist. After this is accomplished, he may feel safe enough with the therapist to develop insights on his own, without benefit of interpretation.

Inferring the Patient's Plan from the First Few Sessions of Therapy

When I was a student at the San Francisco Psychoanalytic Institute, a prominent teacher advised me to avoid formulating the patient's problems, especially at the beginning of treatment. He assumed that in general it is possible to formulate a case only after a prolonged period of exploration, and so that if the therapist develops hypotheses about the patient too early, he risks the premature closure of his mind.

I now believe that this advice is wrong. The therapist should begin during his first contact with the patient to try to understand him. The therapist should attempt to formulate the patient's pathogenic beliefs, his goals, and his plans for working to disconfirm the beliefs and to pursue the goals (Curtis & Silberschatz, 1986; Silberschatz & Curtis, 1986). If the therapist develops explicit (albeit highly provisional) hypotheses about these, he has something to work with. He may check the hypotheses against new observations and thereby confirm them, alter them, or dismiss them. Moreover, the therapist who has in mind the best hypotheses that his current knowledge supports is prepared for the patient's tests, including tests that the patient may give him quite unexpectedly.

During the first few sessions the therapist should try to develop a provisional formulation (theory) specific to the patient. In developing it the therapist relies on information from various sources, including (1) the patient's own formulation of his current problems and goals, (2) the patient's childhood traumas, (3) the therapist's affective responses to the patient, and (4) the patient's reactions to the therapist's approach and interventions.

The therapist may begin to develop his ideas about the patient from one source of information, then check or refine these ideas with information from other sources. *The therapist should not be satisfied with a formulation unless it helps him to understand all or at least most of what he knows about the patient.*

In attempting to determine where the patient wants to go, the therapist is thinking about him in familiar, everyday terms. Unlike the therapist who attempts to infer the patient's impulses and defenses, the therapist who attempts to infer the patient's goals is calling upon well-developed intuitions based on everyday experience. The therapist who is not accustomed to listening for the patient's goals may be surprised to discover how often they are easily perceived. In our research, we have found that judges who are only moderately trained in the present theory can learn to make reliable plan formulations. Moreover, these formulations are valid, as shown by our finding that research relying on them yields a great deal of order (see Chapter 8).

EVALUATING THE PATIENT'S STATED GOALS

In attempting to infer the patient's true unconscious goals from his stated goals, the therapist should assume that the patient's true goals are normal and reasonable. If the patient states implausible goals, he is probably doing so in obedience to powerful unconscious pathogenic beliefs. For example, the therapist should not take at face value a patient's statement at the beginning of treatment that he is interested in a woman who (he implies) is ungiving, demanding, and insulting. The patient's true goal may be to leave her; however, he may be maintaining an attachment to her for various maladaptive reasons. For instance, the patient may believe that he is obliged to suffer in his relations with women as his father suffered in his relations with the patient's mother. Or, if his father failed to protect him from a demanding, vituperative mother, the patient may be testing the therapist in the hope that the therapist will protect him from a demanding, vituperative girlfriend. Or he may be maintaining an attachment to his girlfriend because he believes by leaving her he would destroy her. Or he may be afraid to tell the therapist that he wants to leave his girlfriend, assuming either that the therapist will reprimand him for being selfish or that the therapist will encourage his leaving her before he can tolerate his guilt about doing so.

In some cases, a patient at the beginning of therapy may be unable to state his goals directly. Throughout therapy, but especially at the beginning, he is in unconscious conflict about his wish to reveal his true goals and his fear of doing so. He would like to reveal his goals so that the therapist may help him to pursue them. However, he unconsciously believes that by revealing them he risks being traumatized by the therapist, because he fears that the therapist (whom he has not yet tested) will agree with the pathogenic beliefs that warn him against pursuing his goals.

The degree to which the patient is able at the beginning of therapy to state his true goals varies from patient to patient; it depends, among other things, on the degree to which the patient is bound by his pathogenic beliefs. A patient beginning therapy may be surprisingly insightful about his goals, but may seem to lose his insight soon afterward. At first he may be so powerfully motivated to orient the therapist to his problems that he does so despite his pathogenic beliefs. However, having oriented the therapist, he may soon begin to test him by stating false goals in the hope that the therapist will not take such statements at face value (see Chapter 8 for research supporting this assumption).

In other instances, the patient in his opening remarks may compromise between the wish to reveal his goals and the fear of doing so. For example, a patient who wished to overcome the belief that he should not be proud of his intelligence began the first session by describing himself as a slow learner. However, during the rest of the session he supplied evidence for his in-

telligence by his cogency and clarity in describing his development and his current difficulties.

Another patient who wished to face his drinking problem
and ultimately to stop drinking began his first hour by stating
that he had been nervous about starting therapy, and so drank
a glass of wine the night before. Similarly, a patient who
wanted to convey that he had been unprotected by his parents,
and who hoped in therapy to learn to protect himself, told the
therapist in the first hour that he had gone with an extremely
wild crowd in high school.

In still other instances, the patient may be so afraid to state
his goals that he does not state them at all, or he states goals
opposite to his true goals. However, even in such cases the
patient generally provides some clue as to his true goals. For
example, a man who was fond of his girlfriend unconsciously
believed that his having a successful relationship with her
would show up his mother, who during his childhood frequently told him that no one could get along with him. During
his first few sessions he disparaged his girlfriend as too sweet
and agreeable, and implied that he was considering leaving
her. However, by offering obviously weak arguments for leaving her, he provided the therapist with indirect evidence for his
true goal, which was to develop a close relationship with her.

A patient whose unconscious goals included overcoming
the belief that he should be rejected revealed this goal indirectly
by coolly telling the therapist that he was considering therapy
but was very particular about finding a therapist whom he
considered suitable. He revealed his fear of rejection indirectly
by assuming a rejecting attitude toward the therapist, which
was intended to protect him from the danger of rejection by the
therapist.

In another example, the patient was so endangered by
powerful pathogenic beliefs that she was unable to state any
goal. She suffered a great deal from survivor guilt toward her
emotionally handicapped parents and siblings, and was afraid
that the therapist would agree with her belief that she did not
deserve treatment. In her first few hours she depicted herself as
psychotic and thus as too disturbed for outpatient therapy.
However, she also provided the therapist indirectly with evi-

dence of adequate functioning by the intelligent, organized way that she told her story. She was relieved when the therapist accepted her for treatment. Over a period of time, she revealed both her considerable talents and accomplishments and her concern for her handicapped family. In a sense this patient first conveyed her goal (which was to overcome her survivor guilt) not directly through words, but indirectly through the way she tested the therapist.

EVALUATING THE PATIENT'S CHILDHOOD EXPERIENCES WITH HIS PARENTS

In attempting to understand the patient's problems from a description of his childhood, the therapist is especially interested in determining what traumas the patient suffered in childhood and what pathogenic beliefs he inferred from these traumas. As the therapist comes to understand the patient's pathogenic beliefs, he also comes to understand his goals, which always include disproving these beliefs.

The therapist, in inferring the patient's pathogenic beliefs, should keep in mind that a child tends to take responsibility for the unfortunate things that happen to him and to his family. These include catastrophic events, which give rise to "shock" traumas, and protracted strains resulting from pathogenic relations with parents, which give rise to "strain" traumas.

Shock Traumas

The patient who suffers a sudden catastrophe in childhood tends to experience it as a punishment for something bad he has done. Since he considers it a punishment, he may become unduly guilty, and since he believes himself responsible for it, he may develop a belief in his omnipotence. The more severe the catastrophe, the more guilty and omnipotent he may believe himself to be. In addition, he may infer from the sudden unfortunate turn in his fortunes that catastrophe may strike at any time. He must therefore keep himself vigilant and thus prepared for another blow by fate.

For example, the patient mentioned in Chapter 1 who was sent away from his parents for several months when he was $2\frac{1}{2}$ assumed that he was being punished for demonstrating too much initiative and independence. After the trauma, he became markedly more passive and compliant, and he remained that way into his adult life. He also inferred that he should not be relaxed and happy. During his analysis, whenever he began to feel relaxed, he would warn himself about the danger of relaxation by producing a dream of catastrophe.

A man whose mother died when he was 15 inferred that he had caused her death by his anger toward her. Subsequently, he became quite inhibited in his expression of anger lest he damage the person at whom he was angry. When he came to treatment, he was unable to experience normal anger toward his wife and children.

Harriet A.

Another patient, Harriet A., was severely traumatized when her father deserted the family. He left when the patient was 14 and was killed 2 years later in a car accident. The patient unconsciously took responsibility for her father's departure and death. She assumed that if she had been a better, more loving daughter, her father would have remained in the family and would not have been killed. Before her father's death she had enjoyed life; she was becoming popular in high school and was beginning to date. Harriet unconsciously assumed that her happiness had caused her father's death, and so inferred that she should not be happy, lest she bring about another catastrophe. She suffered a personality change. She became less outgoing. In college she made few friends and spent a great deal of time writing poetry. In her marriage Harriet felt omnipotently responsible for her husband. She tried patiently to satisfy his unreasonable demands and accepted his reprimands submissively. In a long therapy which began when she was 35, Harriet was helped to overcome her pathogenic belief in her responsibility for others. She became more assertive with her husband. She also overcame her survivor guilt to her mother. She ceased being depressed and became more active and outgoing.

A child who is exposed to continuing overwhelming trauma may develop the belief that there is no help for him. He may attempt to ease the pain by withdrawing and anesthetizing himself. For example, a child whose father died when she was 9 was left in the care of her mother, who became depressed and alcoholic. The child felt responsible for her mother. She also felt lonely. She could not talk to her mother or to anyone else about her grief over her father's death. Since the trauma was overwhelming and continuing, she became hopeless and reacted by withdrawing and losing touch with her own affects. In addition, she came to see her family as abnormal and different from the families of her schoolmates. The patient perceived her schoolmates' families as having two happy parents, whereas her family had one depressed parent. She felt ashamed of her family and hence of herself. She tried to deal with this shame by anesthetizing herself to her feelings and attempting to be cheerful and carefree like her schoolmates.

The Child's Compliance with Inadequate Parents

In making inferences about the patient from a description of his childhood, the therapist should keep in mind that the child considers his parents supreme authorities with whom he must get along at almost any cost. He works to develop and maintain his ties to them. He tries to fulfill their expectations and assumes that the ways they treat him are the ways he should be treated. For example, if his parents are rejecting, a child may infer that he deserves to be rejected; his self-esteem may be damaged, and he may believe himself incapable of being loved, not only by his parents but by others.

If the child perceives his parents as depressed, needy, or fragile, he may take responsibility for their happiness and go to great lengths in his efforts to make them happy. For example, a male patient at age 6 became sexually interested in a depressed, languid grandmother. His interest in her was not to gratify himself but to revive her. If a child who believes himself responsible for the happiness of a mother fails in his efforts to make her happy, he may believe himself a failure. A patient whose mother was chronically unhappy and blamed the patient for her unhappiness concluded that he did not deserve to live; he became suicidal.

If a child's parents are unconcerned about him yet demand that he show solicitude and respect to them, he may become depressed, for he may infer that it is his lot to give but not to receive. If a child's parents persistently criticize him for various faults, such as selfishness, arrogance, or stupidity, he may consciously repudiate the criticisms, but unconsciously believe them. As a result, he may come to believe unconsciously that he is not a good person.

If one of the parents is a severe alcoholic, the child is likely to feel both rejected by the parent and worried about him. He may, as a consequence of such trauma, experience a sense of shame. If the family denies the alcoholism, he may experience even more shame. He may also develop the idea that he is not supposed to perceive things as they really are (see Brown, 1985, 1988).

If a child perceives his parents as volatile and capricious—if, for example, they surprise him by unpredictable fits of anger—he may develop the belief that he is always in danger, and so may become hypervigilant. If the child's parents fail to protect him and so expose him to dangers beyond his capacity for coping, he may come to believe that the world is dangerous and that he does not deserve protection. He may become withdrawn or anxious, or subject to attacks of panic (Gassner, 1989).

If the child is sexually abused by a parent, he will blame himself for the abuse and develop a sense of shame. If the parent denies the abuse, the child will infer that he must not remember it. His sense of reality may be impaired. If the abuse occurred at an early age, the child is confronted with the following problem: In order to adapt to his world, he must both forget the abuse and remember it. He must forget the abuse in order to adapt to the members of his family, who insist on denying it, for he cannot be friendly and close to a parent who he knows is abusing him. However, he must remember the abuse in order to prepare for further abuse. If abused while quite young, he may deal with this problem by dissociating, or in certain instances by developing several personalities—one or more of which has no memory of the abuse, and one or more of which remembers it.

The Child's Identifications with Inadequate Parents

In attempting to infer how the patient was affected by his parents, the therapist should keep in mind that for the child his parents are role models. It is from his parents that the child learns how to relate to others. Thus it is extremely difficult for a child to develop abilities that his parents have not developed.

Stuart C.

For example, Stuart C., whose parents had little sense of authority, was himself scarcely able to exert authority. Neither parent could explicitly prohibit him from doing whatever he wanted. His mother could only indicate her disapproval by questioning him. For example, she would ask, "Why do you want to go to the movies?" or "Why do you like to play football?" and so forth. His father would respond to his requests by telling him to ask his mother. In order to protect his parents' authority, Stuart kept himself indecisive. In his adult life he continued to have trouble making and carrying out plans, and, like his parents, was scarcely able to exert authority. In his analysis, Stuart was helped to overcome his indecisiveness. He married, had several children, and became more successful in his work.

Another patient suffered in childhood from parents who were not able to maintain close, satisfactory relations with him. For example, as soon as he and his mother would become involved in a pleasant conversation, she would display discomfort and change the subject or leave the room. His father was even more difficult. He implicitly refused to take the patient seriously; rather, he would tease him by seeming to misunderstand him. As an adult in analytic treatment, the patient noticed that he was uncomfortable when tempted to feel close to another person. For example, he was uncomfortable with women who were respectful and loving. He would become embarrassed and would be tempted to tease them.

If a child perceives his parents as ashamed, he too is likely to develop shame. A patient mentioned in Chapter 2, whose parents revealed their shame about his brain-damaged brother by carefully avoiding any reference to the brother's condition, himself became ashamed of his brother, and ultimately of himself, for coming from a family he considered shameful.

Survivor Guilt

In inferring the patient's pathogenic beliefs from his account of his childhood, the therapist should keep in mind the prevalence of survivor guilt (Modell, 1965, 1971). Most persons suffer from survivor guilt. They assume that in some ways they have been treated better by fate than their parents and siblings, and that their favorable treatment was at the parents' and siblings' expense. A person who suffers from survivor guilt may fail to take advantage of his opportunities, or, if he does take advantage of them, may find some way of punishing himself for doing so.

Survivor guilt may underlie a variety of symptoms. A person who suffers from survivor guilt may torment himself with envy of others who have more than he. By feeling envious, he identifies with his parents and siblings, who (he assumes) are envious of him. Or he may torment himself with shameful ideas, such as that he is absurd, perverted, or unpleasant. He may spoil his relationship with his wife so as not to enjoy a better relationship with her than his parents enjoyed with each other. If his parents were not able to enjoy their children, he may not let himself enjoy his children. If a parent died at an early age, he may become anxious about dying when he reaches that age. If a sibling failed in his career, he himself may become depressed or anxious when he is becoming successful.

Survivor guilt may be both extremely powerful and extremely elusive. A child who grows up in an unhappy family may take unhappiness for granted. He may not realize that even after leaving home he maintains his unhappiness out of loyalty to his family. One patient who became aware of survivor guilt only after considerable work in therapy said, "It was so hard to see because it was like the air I breathe."

A patient may first become aware that he suffers from survivor guilt by inference from experience. He may observe that he develops symptoms either after he is successful or after a close friend or relative suffers a setback. He may only later realize that he feels sorry for certain members of his family and that he considers his advantages unfair. For example, a patient whose parents were extremely anxious when they were away from home developed an embarrassing facial tic whenever he felt adventurous. At first he had no understanding of this symptom. He began to understand it by observing that he developed the tic only when he was enjoying himself in ways his parents could not. It was many months later that he became aware that he felt sorry for his parents in these circumstances.

Separation guilt is also extremely common, if not universal (Modell, 1965, 1971; Loewald, 1979). The patient who suffers from separation guilt believes that if he becomes independent of his parents or siblings, he may upset them. In extreme instances the patient may feel that he has no right to a life of his own. He may, as a consequence of an unconscious belief that he does not deserve to be a separate independent person, convince himself that he enjoys being dependent.

THE THERAPIST'S AFFECTIVE RESPONSES TO THE PATIENT

The therapist, in making inferences about the patient from the ways the patient begins to relate to him, uses his affective reactions as a signal. He senses from his affects how the patient is acting on him, what dangers the patient is warding off, or how the patient is testing him.

Kenneth Y.

During the first few sessions with Kenneth Y., the therapist noticed that he felt himself especially skillful, intuitive, and likable. He inferred from this that Kenneth was unconsciously taking care of him. He assumed that the patient felt omnipotently responsible for others. The therapist's hypothesis was supported by the patient's description of the way he had dealt with his depressed mother. He had bolstered his mother's fragile self-esteem by making himself highly attentive, deferential, and appreciative. The therapist's hypothesis was further supported several weeks later on an occasion when the therapist was late. The patient apparently feared that the therapist would feel guilty, and so was especially ingratiating. In particular, he stated that he had arrived only shortly before the therapist. The therapist reacted by telling Kenneth that he seemed worried about him. Kenneth showed relief and became slightly more straightforward.

In the next example, the therapist used his reactions to the patient during the first hour in making a preliminary formulation of the patient's plan.

Thomas C.

Before his first interview with Thomas C., the therapist heard from the family physician who referred him that Thomas had trouble making himself work. He came from a poor, hard-working family, and both his parents and his wife were worried about his difficulty working. However, during his first session, Thomas, a computer programmer, did not mention his problem about working; indeed, he was relatively uninformative. He chatted informally about various topics. He gossiped about certain mutual acquaintances and talked about the fascinating advances that computers would make possible. He used the therapist's first name and sat in a relaxed posture with his leg over the arm of the chair.

The therapist experienced the patient's casualness as pleasant, confusing, and slightly provocative. He wondered, "Why is the patient so casual? Why is he not talking about his problems?" The therapist was tempted to ask the patient about this. However, he suspected that the patient was being nagged by his parents and wife to work harder, that he probably resented this, and that he was testing the therapist to determine whether the therapist would nag him as they did. Perhaps the patient was struggling to disprove the pathogenic belief that he must at all times be serious, hard-working, and goal-directed.

The therapist therefore decided to reciprocate the patient's casual, friendly attitude; during the first session and throughout the therapy, he refrained from pressing the patient to work in treatment. The patient's response confirmed the therapist's assumption. A few sessions after beginning treatment, Thomas reported that he had tackled a project that he had been avoiding. About a month later he revealed more about his childhood. He stated that his parents had been grim, controlling, and rejecting. As the rest of the therapy confirmed, the patient in childhood had felt both rejected and deprived of autonomy. He now had difficulty working because he experienced work as depriving him of freedom. He was afraid that the therapist would confirm his pathogenic belief that he deserved rejection and did not deserve freedom. He was reassured against this belief by the therapist's response to him. As he realized that the therapist would not try to make him work, he became more able both to relax and to work; his ability to relax and enjoy himself made working feel less burdensome.

In general, if the therapist while listening to the patient feels an unpleasant affect such as confusion, rejection, guilt, or humiliation, he may assume that the patient is turning passive into active.

This may be illustrated by another example, in which a patient during his initial phone call asked the therapist a number of searching questions about his qualifications. During the call the therapist had the unpleasant feeling that unless he was careful, the patient would criticize him. The therapist inferred that in his childhood the patient had suffered hostile criticism from a parent, and that in the phone conversation he was turning passive into active. His assumption proved correct: The patient later reported that his father had been quite critical, and that he (the patient) had been so compliant that he had felt almost paralyzed in his father's presence. He feared that the therapist would criticize him and that he would comply. During the phone call the patient was not only protecting himself from the therapist, but was also testing the therapist's capacity to tolerate being criticized. He unconsciously did not want to commit himself to a therapist who could not stand up to him.

Yet another patient, in his initial phone call, provoked in the therapist a sense of mild bewilderment and rejection. He began in a friendly way by telling the therapist that the therapist was well recommended and by readily setting up a first appointment. However, immediately afterward he began to express grave doubts about the time, effort, and money involved. Like the patient described above, this patient was turning passive into active, both to protect himself from the danger of rejection and to assure himself that the therapist could tolerate the patient's rejecting him.

In the case of Zora T., the therapist, while listening to the patient, had the unpleasant feeling that the patient's problems were almost insuperable.

Zora T.

In her first hour, Zora T., an emigré from Israel, described her situation in bleak terms. She was one of many children whose father had abandoned the family when she was 5 and whose mother died of premature senility at age 38. She was now a widow living alone in a small apartment. She felt weak, had hypertension and asthma, had trouble getting out of bed in the morning, and had no social life. Nor did she get along with two of her three daughters, one of whom was an addict, the other retarded. Several of her grandchildren were not doing well. Her retarded daughter did not know how to mother her own children and would not accept help.

The therapist's initial reaction to Zora's story was to feel burdened. The patient seemed so weighed down with real as opposed to psychological problems that the therapist developed the feeling that he would be unable to help her. He thought to himself, "This patient can't use psychotherapy—she needs money and a good internist."

The therapist inferred from his feeling burdened that Zora might have been severely traumatized in childhood by worry about her overwhelmed, overworked, prematurely senile mother, whom she was unable to help. He assumed too that Zora was testing him, hoping that he would not feel burdened by her. The therapist resisted the temptation to feel burdened, remained upbeat, and accepted the patient for treatment.

The patient's behavior in the next hour tended to confirm the therapist's initial hypothesis. In this hour Zora presented a completely different picture. She was more cheerful. She described her problems at work, where she was in charge of a number of office workers who used computers to process taxes for the federal government. She was the most knowledgeable person there. She resented her boss for ignoring her advice and for taking credit for her work. As she talked, she made it clear that she had an important job, was highly respected, and enjoyed her work.

The rest of her therapy confirmed that Zora's problems stemmed primarily from her relationship to her sick, overburdened mother. (She suffered secondarily from rejection by her father. She hinted at this in the second session in discussing her relationship with her boss.) Zora had believed in childhood that she should relieve her mother of her burdens, and that since she could not do this she was a failure. She also suffered from survivor guilt: She believed that if her mother was so burdened, she herself had no right to be happy. In her first session she tested the therapist by tempting him to feel burdened by her and worried about her, as she had felt with her mother, and she was relieved when he did not do so.

Sometimes the therapist during the first few sessions may find the patient completely opaque. The therapist may be unable to begin to formulate the patient's problems. In these instances the patient may be concealing a shameful secret. He may be so afraid that the therapist will shame him that he adopts a highly defensive posture. He assumes that if he offers the therapist any clues as to the nature of his problem, the therapist will infer his secret and shame him for it.

THE PATIENT'S REACTIONS TO THE THERAPIST

The therapist may check the validity of his ideas about the patient's goals and plans by observing how the patient reacts to him. If the therapist is passing the patient's tests or offering the patient pro-plan interpretations, the patient over a period of time should react favorably. He should demonstrate greater confidence in the therapist, a sense of relief, greater insight, and more boldness. If the patient consistently reacts in these ways, the therapist may assume that he is on the right track and that the formulations on which he bases his behavior with the patient are correct. If the patient consistently fails to respond favorably to the therapist or becomes more depressed and anxious, the therapist may assume that he is on the wrong track.

Sometimes the therapist may gain confidence in his approach when the patient reacts to just a single passed test or a single pro-plan interpretation. This may be illustrated by the case of Kenneth Y., described above. The therapist inferred from his feeling so capable during the first few sessions that Kenneth was unconsciously worried about him and attempting to bolster his (the therapist's) self-esteem. When a few weeks later Kenneth showed relief after the therapist pointed out Kenneth's worry about him, the therapist gained confidence in this inference.

Another example of this occurred early in the therapy of Zora T., the patient who during her first hour described her situation as bleak. The therapist, assuming that Zora was testing him in the hope that he would not feel burdened by her misery, maintained an optimistic attitude. In the next session Zora confirmed the correctness of the therapist's approach by being more cheerful and by revealing that she had an important job and enjoyed her work.

Still another instance occurred early in the therapy of Thomas C., the patient who during the first hour chatted casually with the therapist and offered little or no information about his problems. The therapist inferred that Thomas was testing him in the hope that unlike his stern parents, the therapist would not be worried about his casual approach. The therapist behaved as casually as Thomas. A few sessions later Thomas confirmed the correctness of this approach by reporting that he had begun to work harder, and a month later by revealing that in childhood he had felt constrained by his stern parents.

OTHER CASE EXAMPLES

In the following examples I show how the therapist during the first few sessions develops hypotheses about the patient's plan, including his pathogenic beliefs and his goals.

Janice D.

From the beginning of treatment, Janice D. was aware of some parts of her plan but not of others. Janice, a young woman of Japanese ancestry, began her first session with a female therapist by stating that she was seeking treatment in order to obtain support for her decision not to return to her husband. She continued that her husband was a severe alcoholic, loving when sober but abusive when drunk. He was in Canada, hiding from the police for having killed a man in a drunken brawl. However, he was planning a secret visit home in a few weeks, and Janice feared he would persuade her to return to him.

In her opening remarks, Janice revealed her immediate goal for therapy, but was not conscious of the pathogenic beliefs that she feared would prevent her from realizing it. However, in the first few sessions Janice provided the therapist with enough information to infer one such belief, which was that she deserved to be abused. She stated that she had been severely beaten by both parents from an early age, but only "when I was bad," and also that she had been in numerous affairs with abusive alcoholic men. A few months before she began treatment with her present therapist, Janice had been seeing an elderly male therapist who told her that in her married life she was recreating the experiences of her childhood. She had felt tortured by this therapist and had dreamed that she wanted to kill him. She also had dreamed that she wanted to kill her husband.

From all of this, the therapist inferred the following: Janice had first acquired the belief that she deserved abuse from being abused at an early age by her parents, her first and most absolute authorities. This inference was supported by Janice's statement that her parents only punished her when she was bad, for by this statement she implied that she deserved their punishments. Janice had felt tortured by the previous therapist because she had experienced his interpretations as blaming her for her unhappy marriage, and thus as confirming her pathogenic belief that she had been "bad" and so provoked her husband to mistreat her.

In her dream that she wanted to kill the previous therapist, Janice was telling herself something that she could not quite face in her waking life (see Chapter 7). She had been so compliant to the therapist that she had not let herself become fully conscious that she hated him for implying that she was responsible for her husband's abusing her. It was for similar reasons that she dreamed she wanted to kill her husband. In her waking life, she assumed that she deserved his abuse and so had no right to hate him for it.

The therapist was able to confirm the correctness of the inferences cited above by noting Janice's responses to certain interpretations. Several weeks after the opening sessions, the therapist told Janice that she had been mistreated by her husband and emphasized that she did not deserve this. Janice's immediate response was to become more cheerful and optimistic. That night she dreamed that an old male physician had done a bad job in sewing up her scalp wound, and now a loving nurse practitioner would help her to heal it.

In the session after the dream, Janice showed that she had made good use of her therapist's comments by revealing that in childhood her parents had sometimes beaten her without apparent cause. A week later Janice tested the therapist by appearing to be losing her resolve to stay away from her husband. She stated blandly that she expected to remain friends with him and to see him occasionally. She was immediately relieved when the therapist challenged the wisdom of this plan.

Francine A.

Francine A. was similar to Janice D. in that she came to therapy because she wanted to leave her husband. However, she was unconsciously so guilty about this (she felt omnipotently responsible for her husband's happiness) that she began therapy by stating the opposite—namely, that she wanted to work at improving her marriage. Nonetheless, Francine provided the therapist with considerable indirect evidence for her real goal. Though she tended to blame herself for her unhappy marriage, she indicated by her description of her husband that he was almost impossible to get along with. She depicted him (albeit not explicitly) as not interested in her, and as lazy, passive, ungiving, and blaming.

Francine also gave evidence that she had learned in her childhood relationship with her mother to take a great deal of responsibility for others. She remembered her mother as depressed and demanding. Her mother had expected her to spend a lot of time with her, to cheer her up, and to comfort her. When Francine did not do these things, her mother would accuse her of selfishness, and she would accept her mother's accusations.

From the available evidence, the therapist could not be certain that Francine wanted to get a divorce. However, he inferred that her minimal goals were to stop blaming herself for her marital unhappiness, to see her husband more clearly, and to develop the right to pursue her own interests without believing that to do so was selfish. The therapist received some confirmation of this formulation from Francine's reaction to his first few interpretations. When he pointed out her exaggerated sense of responsibility for her husband, Francine was relieved. A few weeks later, she told the therapist that she wished to devote more time to her oil painting.

Kirsten C.

Kirsten C. began her first session with a tentative statement of her immediate goal, and in addition provided the therapist with enough information to permit him provisionally to infer certain of her pathogenic beliefs. Kirsten began by saying that she had received her M.B.A. a year before. Most of the members of her class now had good jobs, but she was reluctant to look for one. She wondered whether she really wanted to work. Sometimes she thought she did not; other times she thought she did. She did not know why she was reluctant to look for a job. Maybe she was afraid of making mistakes. If a supervisor reprimanded her for an error, she might burst into tears and run out of the room.

At that point, the therapist asked the patient whether she had ever previously behaved in that way. She was silent a minute and then remembered that years before she had felt vulnerable toward her mother. She could not oppose her. She believed whatever her mother told her, even about how she (the patient) felt. For example, the patient had hated summer camp, but she would temporarily believe that she liked it after her mother told her she did.

Later in the same session, Kirsten complained that her parents were not interested in her successes. When she was accepted for the M.B.A. program at Stanford, she telephoned her parents excitedly. Her mother's first reaction was to tell her not to yell into the phone. Later, when in business school, she had been reluctant to discuss her school work with her parents. She thought of the phrase, "I did not want to rub their noses in it." She stated that she was not sure what she meant by that. When encouraged by the therapist to think about it, she stated that neither of her parents had enjoyed their work. She, on the other hand, wanted to be excited about her work. However, her parents would probably disapprove of her feeling excited because it would show them how unlike them she was.

Kirsten added that if she enjoyed her work she would also be different from her younger sister, who had experienced serious problems since her first year of high school. She had done badly in school and been heavily into drugs. Addiction ran in the family. The father was addicted to food and was obese.

From the information offered in the first hour, the therapist inferred that Kirsten had come to therapy because she wanted to get a job. She did not realize how strongly she wanted one, for fear that she would hurt her parents and her sister. She considered her parents weak; in order to protect her mother, she had made herself highly vulnerable to her mother's reprimands. She feared that she would do the same with supervisors at work. She also feared that if she enjoyed work she would hurt her parents and sister by making them envious.

Kirsten felt omnipotently responsible for her parents, suffered from separation/individuation guilt toward her mother, and felt survivor guilt toward her entire family. She was avoiding getting a job in order to protect her parents. This formulation, tentative and general as it was, proved a good guide to technique. As the rest of the therapy demonstrated, it was essentially correct, although incomplete and lacking in detail.

PLANS IN BRIEF TIME-LIMITED PSYCHOTHERAPY

The patients our group studied in brief time-limited (16-session) psychotherapy selected themselves for brief therapy. They responded to an advertisement offering brief therapy to persons who would agree to have their therapies recorded for research purposes. The therapies were to be carried out by experienced therapists at a modest fee.

In the 10 brief therapies I studied informally from transcripts, the patients made limited plans suited to the time limitations of their therapies. Their plans were much more limited than those made, for example, by patients entering analysis. One patient planned to receive help in overcoming her guilt about leaving an abusive spouse. Another patient planned to obtain help in overcoming the separation guilt she felt toward her mother, so that she could obtain a satisfactory job.

During treatment, the brief therapy patient works to carry out his plan in the same ways that the patient in long-term therapy does—that is, by testing his therapist, and by using his interpretations to gain insight into his pathogenic beliefs and goals.

As discussed at greater length in Chapter 8, we used formal quantitative methods to study the therapies of four patients who were treated in brief therapy (Edelstein, 1992; O'Connor, Edelstein, Berry, & Weiss, 1993, in preparation; Weiss, 1993, in press). In each instance, the patient made his plans (goals) clear to the intake worker and then, in the first therapy session, to the therapist. In the following sessions, he seemed to lose insight into his goals, and he also made false (anti-plan) statements about himself. In the middle of his therapy, each of the four patients seemed to lose all insight into his goals. However, toward the end of therapy, the patient once again made his goals relatively clear.

For example, one patient strongly implied during her first session with the therapist that she wished to become less involved with her sick husband and to get a job. Then she began to raise objections to getting a job, claiming that she had never been trained for any sort of work, and thus was unfit to work. Toward the end of therapy the patient again became clear about her wish to obtain a job, and she assumed that she deserved to obtain one. In the last two sessions, she spoke with evident pride about obtaining several interesting jobs.

Our research findings in these four cases strongly support the idea of unconscious planning. Our findings may be explained by the idea that the patient wishes to achieve as much as possible in the time allotted to him. Therefore, in the first therapy session he makes his goals clear to the therapist, so that the therapist can help him to pursue them. Afterward he tests the therapist by seeming to lose insight into his goals or by raising objections to his seeking them, hoping that the therapist will continue to support his pursuit of them. As he gains confidence in the therapist, he tests him more vigorously by losing more insight. Toward the middle of treatment, he appears to lose all insight into his goals. Then, toward the end of his treatment, knowing that he will soon not have a therapist whom he can rely on to pass his tests, he stops testing through losing insight. Indeed, in some instances he tests by acknowledging progress, hoping that his therapist will be pleased by his progress[1]

[1] In a fifth therapy that was studied after this book was written, the patient also lost insight during the course of her therapy. However, a parabolic curve did not significantly fit the raw scores due to greater variability in insight throughout the therapy. The plot of smoothed scores, however, indicated that the pattern was also parabolic, though less dramatically so. The quadratic regression closely approached significance ($p = .052$ for the quadratic term in the regression).

In a study of three brief therapies (Fretter, 1984[2]; Silber-schatz, Fretter, & Curtis, 1986), we demonstrated that the proportion of pro-plan to anti-plan interpretations given to the patient was related to the success of the therapy as determined 6 months after the termination of treatment. The patient who received the highest proportion of pro-plan interpretations did the best. The patient who received the next highest proportion of pro-plan interpretations did the second best. The patient who received the lowest proportion of pro-plan interpretations did the worst.

In the brief therapies that we studied, as in long-term therapies, the patient sets the agenda. In both and long-term therapies the patient, by his statement of his goals at the beginning of treatment and by the ways that he tests the therapist during treatment, permits the therapist to infer how the patient unconsciously wants to be treated, and thus how the therapist may best treat the patient.

---

[2]Fretter's work was supervised by Curtis and Silberschatz.

CHAPTER 5

Testing

Testing is a fundamental human activity prominent in everyday life and in therapy. It is a manifestation of the human being's effort to adapt to his interpersonal world. Through his testing he explores the world to determine its dangers and its opportunities, so that he may protect himself from the dangers and take advantage of the opportunities.

In therapy, the patient tests the therapist from the beginning to the end of treatment. He is vitally interested in finding out how the therapist will react to his plans. Will the therapist oppose his goals, or will he be sympathetic to them and encourage him to pursue them? The therapist's ability to recognize the patient's tests and pass them is central to the therapy. The success or failure of a therapy may depend upon this.

In this chapter on testing, I take up such topics as how the therapist recognizes the patient's tests, how he infers what the patient is trying to find out, how he may know whether he has passed or failed a series of tests, what he should do if he fails the patient's tests, and so forth.

INFERRING HOW THE PATIENT MAY TEST

In inferring how the patient may test him, the therapist, as described in Chapter 4, uses everything he knows about the patient. From this information, he develops a case-specific theory about the patient, which includes the patient's pathogenic beliefs and the goals that the patient has inhibited in obedience to these beliefs. The therapist who has developed a good theory (plan formulation) may check it by assessing its power to explain the patient's ongoing behavior. The therapist may determine whether he is passing the patient's tests by observing the patient's reactions. If he is passing the tests, the patient should react by demonstrating more confidence in the therapist and more movement toward his goals. Also, the patient may bring forth new pertinent information about himself.

In some instances the patient reveals his greater confidence in the therapist by giving him bolder tests. Consider, for example, a patient who believes that his pride will provoke others to put him down, and who tests the therapist by putting himself down in the hope that the therapist will not agree with his self-putdowns. If the therapist consistently refrains from putting him down, the patient not only may become more relaxed and confident in the therapist; he may also test the therapist more vigorously by putting himself down more convincingly than before. He hopes by such testing to garner even greater evidence against his pathogenic beliefs.

The therapist may assume the correctness of his plan formulation, and thus of his understanding of the patient's tests, if his formulation enables him to see the continuity and the coherence of the patient's behavior. The therapist who understands the patient's pathogenic beliefs, tests, and goals perceives in the patient's behavior a coherence and a continuity that the therapist unfamiliar with these concepts cannot perceive. The therapist who subscribes to Freud's 1911–1915 theory is unlikely to realize, when confronted by the patient's varied and shifting affects and behaviors, that the patient is regulating his unconscious mental life throughout therapy in accordance with unconscious plans. Indeed, this therapist may assume that the various fluctuations in the patient's behavior reflect the fluidity of the patient's unconscious mental life.

THE CHARACTERISTICS OF TESTS

Just what patient behaviors should be considered tests is somewhat arbitrary, because tests may differ from other behaviors mainly in degree. Since the patient is interested in the therapist's reactions to everything he says or does, the patient in a sense is always testing the therapist. Moreover, the patient seldom is *simply* testing him; the patient's behavior while testing the therapist invariably serves a variety of other adaptive functions. In testing the therapist, the patient makes use of the events in his everyday life. Suppose, for example, that a patient who fears rejection wants to test the therapist by threatening to stop treatment and hopes that the therapist will urge him to continue. Such a patient may not make this threat until he has a good reason to do so—as when, for instance, he is offered a job in another city. Or a patient who wishes to assure himself that he cannot worry the therapist may not test his potential for worrying him until he suffers a setback in his everyday life that will justify the therapist's worrying. Then he may test the therapist by appearing deeply upset, in the hope that the therapist will not worry unduly.

As implied above, the patient's behavior while testing the therapist may be indistinguishable from his usual behavior. This was the case in the analysis of Roberta P., the lawyer who after 4 years of treatment stated that she wished to terminate in 3 months (see Chapter 3). She made her argument for terminating as plausible as she could. She stated that she had achieved her goals, had developed some friendships, was beginning to date, and was doing better at work. Moreover, she made the reasonable suggestion that she be permitted a period of 3 months before stopping, in which she could focus on her feelings about terminating.

The therapist nonetheless realized that the patient was testing him and that she hoped he would urge her to continue. He based this assumption not on Roberta's behavior, which was indistinguishable from her usual behavior, but on his understanding of her unconscious plan. He knew that she had felt rejected by both parents and that she feared rejection by her colleagues and by the therapist. Also, she had responded favorably to the therapist's attempts to demonstrate acceptance, and her arguments for stopping were weak. She had benefitted from the treatment but was far from having realized her goals.

Moreover, she had no good reason to stop; she had plenty of money and time for the analysis.

In contrast to Roberta's rejection test, some tests are readily recognizable from the way they are presented. The therapist may assume that the patient is testing him in the following circumstances, which are overlapping:

1. The patient behaves in such a way as to arouse powerful feelings in the therapist—for example, by being provocatively boring, contemptuous, seductive, or impossible.

2. The patient exerts a strong pull for the therapist to intervene. He may do this by being silent for long periods of time, by making false or absurd statements, by not paying for some sessions, by feeling highly insulted when the therapist says something clearly intended to be benign, by suddenly threatening in great anger to stop treatment, by insisting the therapist step out of his role as therapist, and so forth.

3. The patient makes use of provocatively wild exaggeration.

4. The patient displays behavior that is out of keeping with his usual behavior, in that it is more foolish or more self-destructive.

In the following example, the patient, William, tested the therapist by forcing him to intervene.

William W.

William W.'s symptoms stemmed from survivor guilt. He believed that whatever successes he achieved were gained at the expense of his parents and sister. The patient was making rapid progress in his second year of treatment when, contrary to his usual behavior, he became provoked when the therapist interrupted him by answering the telephone. He then announced that he was quitting therapy immediately. William apparently had become secure enough with the therapist to risk testing him by behaving unreasonably. His unreasonable behavior served two purposes: to humiliate himself so as to placate his conscience, and to test the therapist in an attempt to assure himself that the therapist could tolerate his successes. When the therapist challenged the patient's wish to stop, the patient felt relieved. He assumed that the therapist approved of his progress, and wished for him to continue making progress.

In the next example, the therapist inferred from the patient's provocative use of wild exaggeration that the patient was testing him.

Arthur D.

In his childhood, Arthur D. had been forbidden by his parents to brag; his parents considered normal self-esteem arrogant. In his therapy, Arthur, who was struggling to overcome the prohibition against pride, tested the therapist by telling him that he had an extremely high IQ. He believed himself to be smarter than almost anyone he knew. He even thought he was one of the smartest persons in the country. Arthur's wild exaggeration had an absurd quality. He used it to put himself down and in addition to test the therapist by offering him an opportunity to put him down, and thus to behave as his parents had.

Also, Arthur assumed that unless he resorted to exaggeration, he would learn nothing new about the therapist. He assumed that a straightforward statement of his abilities—he was indeed intelligent—would not tempt the therapist to question him, and so would not reveal how the therapist felt about his bragging. If he had simply stated that he was highly intelligent, the therapist could scarcely have disagreed.

The therapist passed the patient's test by telling him that he (the patient) was uncomfortable about feeling proud of his high intelligence, adding that for the patient to consider himself intelligent was not arrogant, but was realistic and therefore adaptive.

In the next example, the patient's behavior was readily perceived as testing because it was cruel, foolish, and inconsistent with his usual behavior.

Terry W.

Terry W. had been raised by a lonely, possessive mother and a remote father. His mother, who felt rejected by his father, turned to the patient for companionship. She became so possessive that when the patient left her to play with his friends, she accused him of being cruel. The patient, who consciously dismissed these accusations, unconsciously accepted them.

In his adult life, Terry suffered from the belief that he was responsible for the well-being of others. His main conflict concerned his depressed girlfriend: He wanted to leave her, but was reluctant to do so for fear of hurting her. He felt so uneasy about breaking off the relationship that he delayed telling the therapist that he wanted to break it off. Paradoxically, then, when he informed the therapist of his decision to leave his girlfriend, he pictured himself as motivated by cruelty. He stated that he planned to tell her he was leaving immediately after they had sex, while she was relaxed and affectionate. By this strange plan, which the therapist knew the patient had no intention of carrying out, the patient was complying with his mother's view of him as cruel. He was also testing the therapist to determine whether the therapist would agree with his mother. He was giving the therapist grounds for perceiving him as cruel, hoping, of course, that the therapist would not do so.

The therapist passed the patient's test by telling him that he had a right to leave his girlfriend and that his wish to leave her was not, as he was implying, motivated by cruelty. Rather, it was motivated by the fact that the relationship was not working out for him. The patient was relieved and managed to extricate himself tactfully from his unhappy relationship.

The Patient May Use Different Behaviors to Test the Same Pathogenic Beliefs

The therapist may be helped to understand certain testing sequences by realizing that the patient may use a variety of behaviors to test the same pathogenic beliefs. In one instance, a patient attempted to disprove a particular pathogenic belief by testing it in two seemingly opposite ways. The patient, a young man who wanted to determine whether the therapist was competitive with him, first tested for this by putting himself down. He told the therapist about a blind date in which he had behaved awkwardly and alienated the woman. He hoped unconsciously that the therapist would give no evidence of enjoying his failure. When the therapist did not, the patient felt encouraged; he assumed that if the therapist did not enjoy his failing, he might not object to his succeeding. The patient then tested the therapist by telling him about a success. He described an encounter with a woman who was charmed by him and eager to continue seeing him. The patient hoped that the therapist would give no evidence of being jealous or challenged. When the therapist did not, the patient felt relieved and told the therapist more about his comfort with women.

In the following example, too, the patient used different kinds of behaviors in an attempt to disprove the pathogenic belief that the therapist was not interested in her except for his own selfish purposes.

Valerie T.

The patient, Valerie T., a woman in her 30s, taught chemistry at a local university. From the beginning of therapy, she unconsciously feared that the therapist would reject her. Soon after she began therapy, she attempted to assure herself against this danger by giving the therapist a rejection test. She told him that she was considering a teaching position in a university outside the area. Valerie was relieved when the therapist questioned the wisdom of her doing this, pointing out that she had a good job locally and had just begun her therapy. She felt reassured for a while. However, her fear of rejection soon came back in a new form: She began to fear that the therapist was seeing her not primarily for her sake, but because he found her sexually attractive. She now tested him by being seductive. On one occasion she suggested that since the weather was good, they have their session in the park a few blocks from the office. When the therapist did not respond to the patient's seductiveness, she gained confidence in him and began gradually to investigate the problem that had brought her into therapy—namely, her difficulty getting along with her colleagues.

The Therapist May Sometimes Understand the Meaning of a Test Only After He Has Passed It and the Patient Has Brought Forth New Material

In most therapies, there are times when the therapist knows he is being tested but does not know just what pathogenic beliefs the patient is attempting to disprove. In such circumstances, the therapist may not know whether he has passed the patient's tests until the patient responds. If the patient reacts to the therapist's interventions by retreating, the therapist may assume that he has failed the tests. If the patient moves forward, he may that assume that he has passed the tests. If the therapist passes the tests and the patient responds favorably, the therapist may infer from the nature of the patient's responses just what pathogenic beliefs the patient was working to disprove.

In the following example, a patient gave her therapist a powerful test. The therapist did not fully understand the meaning of the test until he passed it and the patient brought forth pertinent new material that opened a new chapter in the therapy.

Nancy C.

The patient, Nancy C., a physician in her mid-30s, came to treatment primarily because she was concerned about how she was behaving with her husband. She would become enraged at him and hit him, sometimes without much provocation. During her first few therapy sessions, Nancy had difficulty talking; she was impeded by an intense sense of shame about herself and her parents. She was especially upset while describing her relations with her mother, who was easily hurt, had a violent temper, and during her childhood frequently beat her. Nancy scarcely mentioned her father except to say that she was fond of him.

Throughout the first 18 months of therapy, the patient made steady progress. She was able by testing the therapist to assure herself that she could not easily provoke him, that he would not shame or reject her, and that it was relatively safe for her to be fond of him. In addition, she began to get along better with her husband. Then the therapy was unavoidably interrupted: The therapist, as he had told the patient well in advance, had to be out of town for 4 months. Before he left, he arranged at the patient's request for her to continue treatment with a colleague while he was gone.

When the patient resumed therapy after the 4 months' interruption, she immediately informed the therapist that she planned to reduce the frequency of her sessions from twice a week to once a week, and, in addition, to continue treatment once a week with the second therapist. The first therapist, who assumed incorrectly that Nancy was giving him a rejection test, urged her to resume seeing him twice a week and to stop seeing his colleague. However, he soon discovered that the patient had no intention of doing this, and so he accepted the new arrangement. A few weeks later the patient surprised the therapist with a new disclosure: In her childhood she had been not only physically abused by her mother, but also sexually abused by her father. She was upset describing the abuse. She felt guilty and ashamed. She suffered most acutely from a sense of disloyalty to her father. Nancy had been fond of her father and had experienced him as more reliable than her mother; moreover, he had sworn her to secrecy.

At this point it became clear why, after the 4 months' interruption, the patient had insisted on the new arrangement. It was to give the therapist a powerful transference test. Nancy defied the therapist's wish in a way that she considered highly disloyal. She thereby risked losing a relationship that was important to her, for she loved the therapist and had been helped a great deal by him. When the therapist passed this test by maintaining his usual relationship with the patient, Nancy came to realize that the behavior she considered disloyal was not so dangerous, either to herself or to the therapist. She then felt it safe to do something she considered disloyal to her father—namely, to defy him by describing his abusing her. As the patient came to face the abuse directly, she no longer had a need to continue with the second therapist, and she resumed twice-a-week therapy with the first.

In the next example, the therapist did not even know he was being tested until the patient made this evident by the new material that she produced.

Darlene S.

Darlene worked excessively hard at her job and had no time for recreation. However, she did not seem to consider this a problem. Then, during a session in her second year of therapy, she made it clear that she was making progress in becoming less ascetic. She announced that she had decided to leave work earlier and perhaps take longer vacations. Darlene then added that the therapist did not seem to be exerting himself very much during their sessions. Only then did the therapist become aware that Darlene had been testing him. She had been subtly pressuring him to work harder by complaining about her slow progress, and he had passed her tests by remaining relaxed.

By pressuring the therapist, the patient was presenting him with passive-into-active tests. In her childhood both her parents had worked all the time, and they seemed uncomfortable when Darlene was not working. They would point out the various tasks that she had not yet completed. Darlene had been doing this to the therapist and was relieved when the therapist did not respond to her pressure. She could now use the therapist's example in her struggle against the pressure of her internalized parents.

In the next example, the therapist rather abruptly changed his tack with the patient, and the patient's extremely favorable response to the change threw a great deal of light on how the patient wanted the therapist to treat her.

Margaret M.

Margaret M., a 70-year-old schizophrenic woman, suffered from auditory hallucinations and paranoid ideas. The patient was one of nine children of poor immigrant farmers. She was severely deprived in childhood: Although she received little parenting, she tried to take care of her overburdened mother and of several younger siblings who were put in her charge. In her therapy, in which she was seen for 20 minutes a week (she would become uncomfortable after 20 minutes), Margaret's speech was vague and incoherent. She was preoccupied with her paranoid ideas and with her fear that, because the state was paying for her therapy and for other medical expenses, she was receiving more than her due. She implied that because of this fear, she was having difficulty continuing therapy. The therapist felt under some pressure to alleviate her worries.

The therapist in fact had received no payments from the state for a long time, because it cost him more to bill for the patient's brief visits than he would have received in payment. He had been reluctant to tell this to the patient, for fear she would assume she was cheating him. However, eventually the therapist responded to the patient's pressure by changing his mind. He told her that from then on he would see her free of charge, thereby making it unnecessary for the state to pay for her visits.

The patient seemed reassured. In the next session, for the first time in her long therapy, Margaret reported a dream. Moreover, in contrast to her usual productions, the dream was well constructed, vivid, and dramatic. The patient dreamed that she was in a small wooden hut by herself on a plain. A storm raged outside, and the ground around the hut was covered with deep snow. The patient heard a thud outside and was sure that it was caused by her mother falling down in the snow. She rushed to the door, opened it, and was relieved that no one was there.

The therapist assumed that in the dream Margaret was telling herself that she did not have to take care of her mother. Apparently the patient had been strongly affected by the therapist's offer to see her free of charge. This permitted her to experience herself as someone who had a right to receive from others, rather than as someone who had to take care of others. The patient's dream made the therapist aware that by giving her free treatment he was helping her to overcome the belief that she was undeserving. He began to give the patient small inexpensive presents from time to time, which she enjoyed receiving and which helped her to feel a little more self-esteem and a little less worry about others.

TESTING WITH ATTITUDES

In some therapies the patient gives the therapist sharply defined, powerful tests. This was the case in the therapy of Roberta P., the lawyer who after 4 years of only modestly successful analysis announced that she planned to terminate in 3 months. This was also the case in the therapy of Nancy C., who, after her therapist's 4-month leave of absence, insisted on continuing once a week with the therapist she had been seeing while he was gone.

In contrast, there are therapies in which the patient, instead of attempting to disprove his pathogenic beliefs by discrete tests, attempts to disprove them by displaying a persistent attitude that serves the same testing function. For example, a patient may work to disprove the belief that if he is friendly he will be rejected. He may test it with occasional discrete displays of affection, or he may attempt to accomplish the same thing by displaying a persistently friendly attitude. The therapist, in treating such a patient, should develop an attitude toward him that is designed to help the patient disprove his pathogenic beliefs. For example, in treating a patient who displays a persistently friendly attitude in order to test the belief that he should be rejected, the therapist should return the patient's friendliness.

A good example of a patient who tested by the display of a particular attitude is the computer programmer, Thomas C., discussed in Chapter 4. Thomas had inferred from the constraints imposed on him during his childhood that he was supposed to have little freedom or fun; rather, like his mother, father, and siblings, he should be working most of the time. In the therapy he tested this belief by persistently displaying a conspicuously casual attitude. He made no pretense of working in therapy, and unconsciously hoped that the therapist would not try to make him work. The therapist responded to the patient by being casual and relaxed himself and by not pressuring the patient to work. Thomas was relieved. The therapist's acceptance of his relaxed, casual approach helped him to realize that he unconsciously felt under a great deal of pressure to work. He began to let himself have more fun and freedom in his everyday life. He also began to do much better at his job: Knowing that he did not have to work all the time, he was able to work hard some of the time. In addition, he remembered more about the sense of constraint he had suffered as a child.

Another example of testing with attitudes occurred in the therapy of Leonard Y.

Leonard Y.

Leonard Y. had felt rejected by his parents and assumed that he deserved the rejection. In his therapy, he worked to disprove this belief by being persistently friendly. The therapist responded by returning Leonard's friendliness. During some sessions the patient and therapist simply chatted in a casual, relaxed way about various events and problems in the patient's life. However, every once in a while Leonard would remember childhood episodes in which he had felt rejected by his parents. For example, on several occasions he remembered instances of his mother's ignoring him in favor of his older brother, or of his father's responding to his attempts to talk about problems by giving him lectures on morality.

In his occasional interpretations, the therapist elaborated on the patient's comments. He helped the patient to realize that he had experienced his parents as rejecting, that he had believed he deserved their rejection, and that this belief was false and a poor guide in his present life. Over a period of 4 years, Leonard benefited a great deal from his therapy. He became more comfortable with friends, developed the courage to date, and eventually developed a satisfactory long-term relationship with a woman.

Leonard worked in therapy by displaying a transference attitude. He had learned in childhood that if he was friendly to his parents he risked rejection, and he tested this belief by a display of friendliness to the therapist. In the next example, the patient, Stephan X., tested his pathogenic beliefs not by a transference attitude but by a passive-into-active attitude. That is, he behaved toward the therapist as his parents had behaved toward him.

Stephan X.

Stephan X. had experienced his parents as never satisfied with him, and he had complied with their dissatisfaction by considering himself defective. The patient worked in therapy by displaying a passive-into-active attitude in which he was dissatisfied with the therapist as his parents had been dissatisfied with him. He hoped that the therapist would not feel put down by him, so that he could use the therapist as a model in fighting his compliance with his parents' dissatisfaction.

In the therapy, Stephan often appeared dissatisfied with the therapist and the therapy. He would respond to the therapist's comments with sighs and grimaces. The therapist persistently resisted feeling put down by the patient, and in a matter-of-fact way, he fought back against the patient's apparent displeasure. He asked the patient why he was disgruntled, and he did not accept the patient's accusations.

Stephan would remain petulant for long periods of time, during which he would display little or no insight. Then every once in a while he would bring forth new material that illuminated his behavior. For example, he remembered instances when he had tried to please his parents and his parents had ignored or ridiculed him. The therapist, by his few interpretations, helped the patient to realize that he had inferred from his relations with his parents that he could not please them or others. Stephan made progress: He developed the capacity to stand up to critics, became less shy at work, and became better able to counter his wife's complaints about him.

DISCRIMINATING BETWEEN TRANSFERENCE TESTS AND PASSIVE-INTO-ACTIVE TESTS

The therapist may sometimes distinguish predominantly transference tests from predominantly passive-into-active tests by the way he experiences the patient's testing behavior. When the patient transfers, he endows the therapist with the authority of a parent, so the therapist tends to feel relatively safe. However, when he turns passive into active, the patient assumes the role of the traumatizing parent, and the therapist may feel considerable strain. Thus, if the therapist experiences the patient's behavior as confusing, worrisome, outrageous, frightening, or impossible, or if the therapist finds himself feeling guilty, the patient is usually giving a passive-into-active test. (He may also be transferring.)

The fact that the tests most disturbing to the therapist are almost always passive-into-active tests may be understood in terms of the difference between the relationship of the child to his parent and that of the parent to his child. As I have noted throughout this book, the child is powerfully motivated to maintain his ties to his parents; for the child to do this is a matter of life and death. The child is so highly motivated to get along with his parents that he will not behave outrageously unless he does so in compliance with his parents, or through identification with his parents' outrageous behavior.

However, some parents are not highly motivated to maintain their ties to their child or to get along with the child. Sometimes a parent may abandon, beat, worry, or seduce a child. Thus if a therapist feels quite belittled by a patient, guilty to him, confused or humiliated by him, or helpless to treat him, the patient is almost always behaving like a parent—and thus turning passive into active.

In the following example, the therapist was able to distinguish the patient's passive-into-active tests from her transference tests by the way he felt while being tested. When the therapist experienced the patient's demands as extremely disagreeable, he assumed correctly that she was turning passive into active. When he experienced her demands as reasonable, he assumed correctly that she was transferring.

Lisa O.

The patient, Lisa O., suffered from two powerful pathogenic beliefs. First, she believed herself omnipotently responsible for others and compelled to comply with them lest she hurt them. Second, she believed that she did not deserve help and so could get no one to satisfy her wishes. In therapy, the patient used the same behavior to test both beliefs in the hope of disproving them: She urgently requested the therapist to offer her extra hours. At first she made her requests in a very disagreeable way, and the therapist inferred from this that Lisa was testing him by turning passive into active. Lisa unconsciously wanted the therapist to refuse her so that she could learn from him how to say "no." The therapist refused the patient's requests, and the patient benefited. Gradually, over a period of several years, Lisa became more relaxed, stronger, more able to avoid complying with others, and more aware of the belief (and its irrationality) that if she did not comply with others she would hurt them.

After several years of therapy, Lisa changed the way in which she requested an extra hour: She behaved as though she really wanted an extra hour. Accordingly, the therapist now began to experience her requests not as provocative but as genuine. He assumed that the patient might now be testing him to disprove her belief in her helplessness. After the therapist granted the first extra hour, the patient was more relaxed than usual and brought forth a new memory. It was of an event when she was 8, shortly after her mother's sudden death. She was lying in bed trying to wish her dead mother back to life and feeling helpless that she could not do so.

Apparently Lisa was now indeed testing to disprove the belief that she was unable to summon help. When the therapist granted her the extra hour, she felt a little less helpless. This made it possible for her to remember an occasion when she was overwhelmingly helpless. When the patient called and the therapist came, the patient felt better, and was able to remember an occasion when she had called and her mother did not come.

The order in which Lisa chose to work at disproving her pathogenic beliefs was dictated by considerations of safety. At the beginning of therapy she was unconsciously quite frightened by her expectation, based on a fear of hurting the therapist, that she would have to comply with him and accept false interpretations or follow bad advice. Therefore, soon after starting therapy, she began to work at changing her belief that unless she complied with the therapist she would hurt him. She made demands on the therapist in a disagreeable way, hoping that he would refuse them so that she could identify with his capacity to do this. The therapist did refuse them, and the patient, over a period of time, acquired the capacity to say "no." As she overcame her fear of complying with the therapist, she could let herself experience a strong need for him. It was then that her request for extra hours began to sound genuine.

A patient who could not learn from his parents how to deal with a particular kind of trauma may turn passive into active in order to learn from the therapist how to deal with it. Consider, for example, a patient who could not tolerate being criticized. He was so compliant to criticisms that at times he felt completely unable to counter them. He had developed this problem in childhood in relation to parents who, though quite critical of him, were themselves unable to tolerate criticism from him. The patient believed he had to accept his parents' criticisms lest he hurt them. In his therapy he tested the therapist by criticizing him, often vehemently, hoping that he would not upset the therapist or that the therapist would fight back, so that he could learn from the therapist how to tolerate criticism and how to fight back.

A patient is likely to turn passive into active if in childhood he complied with parental mistreatment, but did not realize either in childhood or in later life that his parents' treatment of him was unreasonable. A patient may not realize how badly his parents treated him if he was socially isolated and so had no opportunity to observe normal parent–child relations. A patient such as this may be afraid of transferring; he may fear that the therapist will mistreat him in the same ways his parents mistreated him. However, he may feel no compunction about turning passive into active. Since he believes that his parents' traumatizing behavior was justified, he is likely to feel somewhat justified in repeating such behavior with the therapist.

There are exceptions to the rule that the patient whose requests are burdensome or extremely difficult to satisfy is turning passive into active. A patient who has been severely deprived, or who has been criticized by his parents for making reasonable requests, may make burdensome demands in order to give transference tests. He may stridently request extra hours or the right not to pay for several missed sessions, in the hope that the therapist will not be burdened by him or critical of him, as his parents were. The therapist may help the patient who tests in this way by attempting to grant his requests, or, if he cannot grant them, by telling the patient that he deserves to have them granted but that he (the therapist) is not in a position to do this.

TESTING BY TURNING PASSIVE INTO ACTIVE

Most patients, but not all, test by turning passive into active at some time during their therapies. Some patients do so only occasionally, in response to particular traumatic events or in preparation for difficult challenges. Others do so frequently throughout their treatments.

A patient who is struggling with powerful affects that he cannot master may work to master them by turning passive into active. For example, a female patient whose mother and sister were both dying tragic deaths was overwhelmed with sadness that she could scarcely face. In her therapy, she tested the therapist by describing her mother's and sister's situations in such poignant terms that the therapist felt like weeping. The patient was helped to tolerate her sadness by identifying with the therapist's capacity to tolerate sadness.

A patient in therapy who experiences intense guilt about his wish to oppose a parent may give the therapist a passive-into-active test, which the therapist may pass by displaying an ability to oppose the patient. Consider, for example, a female patient whose father abused her and at the same time denied he was doing so. The patient unconsciously wished to expose her father, but was prevented from doing this because she considered exposing him disloyal. In therapy the patient told the therapist about the abuse, then tested him by telling him that it really did not happen. The therapist passed this test by telling the patient that he believed she had been abused but was uncomfortable about acknowledging it. The therapist's ability to challenge the patient's denials helped the patient to challenge her father's denials.

A patient who is planning to take a certain initiative but is unsure about how to carry it out may prepare for it by giving the therapist passive-into-active tests. Through such tests, the patient attempts to present the therapist with the same kind of problem that he expects to face; he hopes to learn from the therapist how to handle this kind of problem. Below, I present several examples of this type of passive-into-active testing, beginning with the case of Gina H.

Gina H.

Gina H. suffered from a mild depression, which stemmed in part from the pathogenic belief that she was a bad person and a failure because she could not keep her depressed mother happy. A few months after she began therapy, she casually discussed with the therapist the pros and cons of the therapist's giving her antidepressant drugs. After she established that the therapist had no intention of giving them to her, she started demanding them in an obnoxious way. She insulted the therapist, calling him stubborn and stupid. When the therapist continued to refuse her, she consulted a specialist in psychopharmacology. She persuaded the consultant to call the therapist and suggest antidepressants. However, the therapist continued to refuse.

Finally, after several weeks, Gina relented. Soon afterward, she told the therapist that she had been quite anxious about her upcoming trip home to see her mother. She was worried that she would feel helpless around her mother and compelled to do whatever her mother asked her to do.

Gina had been preparing for her trip home by testing the therapist. She had been giving him the same kind of problem that she expected to face. She demanded antidepressant drugs in the hope that the therapist would refuse her, so that she could learn from his example how to refuse her mother. She was sufficiently strengthened by the therapist's example that she could deal with her problem with her mother directly. This was a step forward. It led to Gina's becoming aware of her great sense of responsibility for her mother, and of her fear that if she refused her mother she would upset her a great deal.

Felice M.

Another example of a patient preparing for a challenge by passive-into-active testing occurred in the analysis of a young woman, Felice M. She wanted to leave her demanding boyfriend but felt guilty about doing so, for she knew he would feel rejected. Felice worked to gain the courage to leave him by testing the analyst, who she knew would object to her wanting to reduce the frequency of her sessions from four to three times a week. After giving extremely weak arguments for cutting back, Felice insisted somewhat obnoxiously for several months that she be allowed to cut back.

The analyst tried to investigate the patient's motivations, but Felice refused to discuss them. At one point, uncertain about the nature of the patient's tests, the analyst softened his stand by show-ing a slight willingness to consider the patient's request. Felice appeared alarmed and behaved as though she had not heard what the analyst said. This convinced the analyst that the patient wanted him to stick to his guns, and he did so. He assumed that the patient was made quite uncomfortable by the prospect of his giving in, for if he gave in, she would be unable to use him as a model in her struggle to maintain her stand with her boyfriend. Felice chose to ignore the analyst's wavering, hoping unconsciously that he would feel coached by this to maintain his stand.

Felice resumed her demands by complaining self-righteously that the analyst was forcing her to accept a unilateral decision which she insisted should have been discussed further with her. Eventually she made it clear that she herself was preparing to make a unilateral decision—namely, to leave her boyfriend. She had been helped to take this step by the analyst's example.

Gloria S.

Still another example of the use of passive-into-active testing to prepare for an upcoming task occurred in the analysis of a young woman, Gloria S., who suffered from an exaggerated need to please others. She developed the belief that unless she pleased others she would hurt them. She developed this belief in her relations with her parents, who were demanding, and deeply upset whenever she refused their requests.

Throughout most of her analysis, Gloria tested this pathogenic belief. She made numerous demands on her female analyst for such things as a longer hour, a reduction in fee, extra hours, and so forth. She threatened to feel deeply hurt if the analyst refused such demands; however, she usually seemed strengthened by her refusing them. Over the first few years of analysis, she was helped by working in this way. She became better able to stand up to her parents and friends.

During the third year of analysis, the patient's mother died in an automobile accident on the very day that the patient's Ph.D. dissertation was accepted by her committee. Gloria had expected to have her mother read the dissertation. Now, overwhelmed with grief, she gave it to her analyst, poignantly demanding that she read it. During the same session the patient discussed her worry about her father, who lived in another part of the country. She knew he would feel bereft by her mother's death. She feared that he would expect her to move home with him to take her mother's place.

The next session, after investigating the patient's expectation that she would read the dissertation, the analyst returned it unread. The analyst, by returning the dissertation, passed an important passive-into-active test. Gloria feared that she would be compelled by her father's intense grief to stay home with him and take his wife's place. When she observed that the analyst did not feel compelled by her grief to read the dissertation and thus to take her mother's place, she felt supported against her father's demands. When she returned home for her mother's funeral, she was able to be loving with her father and yet to refuse a prolonged visit with him.

The three examples presented above demonstrate that to pass certain tests, the therapist may have to refuse an apparently reasonable request. This is worth emphasizing because some therapists, perhaps misunderstanding Kohut's views about empathy, assume that whenever the patient makes a reasonable request the therapist should grant it. Just how the therapist should respond to a request varies from patient to patient, depending on his understanding of the patient's unconscious plan. Sometimes when the therapist persistently grants the patient's requests, he fails the patient's tests, and the patient becomes progressively worse. A patient who unconsciously has a powerful need to learn from the therapist how to say "no" may make progressively more outlandish requests, in the hope that he can force the therapist to refuse him.

However, as noted above, there are numerous instances in which the therapist in order to pass the patient's tests, should go along with him. In such instances the therapist by refusing the patient's requests so as to follow the rule of abstinence may be quite harmful.[1] An example of this occurred in the therapy of Lisa O., reported earlier, who benefited when the therapist granted her request for an extra session. She remembered her vain attempts to wish her mother back to life. This patient was enabled to remember her longing for her mother not by the therapist's frustrating her request for an extra session, but by his acceding to this request, thereby helping her feel safe enough to retrieve the painful memory.

TESTING THAT DISTURBS THE THERAPIST

This section is concerned with patients whose testing disturbs the therapist. Among these are patients who are extremely insulting; patients who frequently take offense and blow up angrily at remarks obviously intended to be benign; patients who, while seeming to benefit from therapy, complain that the therapist has ruined their lives; patients who complain bitterly about the therapist's ineffectiveness while telling the therapist nothing about themselves; patients who repeatedly imply that unless the therapist is more helpful they will kill themselves, patients who persistently refuse to pay for certain hours in which they claim to have received no help; patients who with no cause threaten to sue the therapist for malpractice, patients who unjustifiably give the therapist the feeling that he is making serious mistakes; and so forth.

---

[1]In his 1911–1915 theory, Freud wrote that the therapist should not be too gratifying to the patient. He referred to this principle as the rule of abstinence.

In general, therapists should not try to treat more than one or two such patients at a time, for they require much time and effort. Moreover, a therapist who is especially uncomfortable with such patients should not try to treat them. However, in sending such a patient away the therapist should not imply that he is untreatable, for the patient may be helped by a therapist who is comfortable with him and who knows how to treat him.

The patient who disturbs the therapist is almost always turning passive into active; that is, he is testing the therapist by behaving as a parent or older sibling behaved toward him. He hopes that the therapist will not be crushed by his behavior as he was crushed by a parent's or sibling's behavior. In most instances the patient is also transferring. For example, the patient who threatens the therapist, or who disturbs everyone in the building by screaming and slamming doors, is both turning passive into active and transferring. He is implicitly asking the therapist to set some kind of limit; he also hopes that despite his disturbing behavior, the therapist will not reject him by giving up on him.

The therapist who realizes that the patient who disturbs him is working by testing him may be in a better position to help the patient than is the therapist who assumes that the patient is being obnoxious, vile, or destructive simply to gratify himself. It is easier for a therapist both to respect a patient and to empathize with him when he realizes that the patient, through his disturbing behavior, is working to overcome his problems. Moreover, the idea that the patient is testing alerts the therapist to a way of helping the patient—that is, by passing his tests—and so may protect the therapist from discouragement.

In treating such a patient, the therapist tries to figure out how he is being tested. He attempts to infer this from everything he knows about the patient, including the patient's account of how he behaved toward his parents and how his parents behaved toward him. The therapist also relies heavily on his affective responses to the patient. Often he may infer from the way he feels when he is with the patient how the patient felt when he was with his parents. The therapist may tentatively assume that if he feels helpless, defeated, extremely anxious, overly responsible, or intensely guilty, the patient felt that way toward a parent. For example, the therapist who during his first session with Zora T. felt that her problems were insuperable (see Chapter 4) inferred from this that Zora in childhood might have felt burdened by her sad mother and guilty that she could not make her mother happy.

The therapist who feels that unless he is extremely careful with his patient he will make a serious mistake may be reacting to passive-into-active omnipotence tests, which the patient hopes will not induce the therapist to worry inappropriately. Thus the therapist who feels he must be extremely careful with his patient may tentatively infer that the patient felt an omnipotent sense of responsibility for a parent about whom he worried a great deal.

As another example, consider the patient who professes envy of the therapist and who induces the therapist to feel guilt about being better off than the patient. The patient is probably giving the therapist a passive-into-active survivor guilt test, and the patient hopes that the therapist will not be upset by the patient's envy. The patient may then, by identifying with the therapist, become less concerned about a parent's envy of him. To give still another example, the therapist who feels quite worried about leaving a patient when he takes a vacation may be reacting to passive-into-active tests by which the patient hopes to disprove a belief that he (the patient) should feel guilty when leaving a parent.

In order to pass the patient's passive-into-active tests, the therapist tries to demonstrate a better way of dealing with the patient's disturbing behavior than the patient used in childhood to deal with his parents' disturbing behavior. The therapist's approach and attitude are as important as his interpretations, if not more so. In general, the therapist should not interpret the patient's disturbing behavior as soon as he displays it. Before he interprets it, he should attempt to demonstrate that he is able to deal effectively with it. Suppose that a patient identified in childhood with an unhappy, blaming mother, and complains in therapy about how depressed he feels and how little the therapist is helping him. In general, the therapist should not attempt to explain the patient's blaming him by pointing to his identification with his blaming mother until he has demonstrated that he can tolerate the patient's misery and blame. If the therapist interprets this identification before demonstrating that he can tolerate the blame, the patient may assume that the therapist is blaming him in order to protect himself. The therapist may appear defensive to the patient, and thus may fail to provide the patient with a good model of how to deal with his mother's disturbing behavior.

The therapist may sometimes be thrown off course by disturbing accusations. If the therapist recovers and deals effectively with these, the therapist's temporary upset does no harm. Indeed, the patient may be reassured by it: He may realize that the therapist is not glib or overly defended, and that even if upset by the patient's accusations he may recover and behave appropriately. The patient then, by using the therapist as a model, may learn that he too may become upset and then recover.

When the therapist does begin to make interpretations to the disturbing patient, he should be concerned not only with the content of his interpretations, but also with his attitude while delivering them. For example, if the patient is giving the therapist passive-into-active worry tests, the therapist may detract from a good interpretation by delivering it in a tense, worried manner.

This may be illustrated by the therapy of a female patient who in childhood had worried a great deal about her chronically ill father. She felt it was her job to keep him alive. She reminded him to take his medicines, and she observed him carefully to evaluate his state of health. In therapy, the patient tested the belief that she was responsible for others by turning passive into active. She behaved as though the therapist was responsible for her welfare. The therapist began to interpret the patient's fear that the therapist would worry about her as she had worried about her parents. For a number of weeks this interpretation was not helpful. Then the therapist realized why it was not: He had unconsciously accepted the patient's invitation to be omnipotent. He was trying too hard to be helpful, and thus was delivering his interpretations in an intense, worried style. When he realized his mistake, he changed and began to offer his interpretations in a relaxed style. He simply floated interpretations by the patient. The patient appeared relieved and began to do better.

A patient may find the interpretation of his disturbing behavior quite helpful. He may not understand why he is disagreeable, and he may feel quite guilty about being that way. He may be greatly relieved when the therapist demonstrates an understanding of his behavior by telling him, for example, that out of loyalty to a parent he is imitating the parent, or that he is re-enacting childhood traumatic experiences with a parent and taking the parental role, or that he is attempting to show the therapist how he felt as a child. The patient may be relieved to realize that his behavior does not derive from inherently bad impulses, and that he is not being frivolous, self-destructive, or wanton simply to gratify himself. Rather, his behavior derives from childhood identifications with a traumatizing parent, and he is working in therapy to understand his childhood traumatic experiences and to disprove the pathogenic beliefs inferred from them. These points can be illustrated by the example of Walter A.

Walter A.

Walter A., a young man, repeatedly criticized his young male therapist. Walter told the therapist over and over again that he wasn't helpful; that he didn't know what he was doing; that he didn't have enough experience to be helpful; that he was bewildered, confused, repetitive, and banal; and so on. The therapist responded by being calm and reassuring. Finally, after demonstrating that he could tolerate the patient's vitriol, the therapist said, "I think maybe you're trying to show me how you felt with your family when you were growing up. Maybe your father was critical and put you down over and over again." The patient answered immediately, "No, it was my older sister. I'd be watching TV and she would hit me repeatedly on the face. I would sit very still, because I thought that if I moved she would become more vicious. She would call me 'stupid,' and 'dumb.'" Walter then broke into tears and wept for the rest of the hour. He felt relieved. He was able to sympathize with himself instead of seeing himself as a vicious, ungrateful man. He realized that he had been criticizing the therapist not from primary hostility, but as part of his working in therapy. Moreover, he realized that he had been severely traumatized by his older sister's abuse of him.

A somewhat similar example concerns a patient who dismissed everything the therapist said; she called it useless, stupid, repetitive, and so on. Moreover, she frequently threatened to leave treatment. After tolerating this for some time, the therapist finally said, "Perhaps you're behaving toward me as your mother behaved toward you, and you're afraid I'll be upset by you as you were by your mother." The patient agreed and became sad. She also began to mimic the shrill, petulant voice that her mother used when criticizing her. The patient, though relieved, soon resumed her passive-into-active testing, and she continued to work mainly in this way for several years. However, as illustrated above, she would occasionally pause and remember some of the traumatic experiences she was re-enacting with the roles reversed. During the last year of her therapy, the patient became more reasonable. She then began to feel sorry for her mother, whose nasty behavior made it impossible for her (the mother) to maintain good relationships with friends or family. This threw light on another function of the patient's disagreeable behavior—namely, to protect herself from survivor guilt.

In treating the patient who is insulting and blaming, it may be important for the therapist to demonstrate a variety of reactions. For example, the therapist should at times fight back against obviously unfair or extravagant or foolish accusations, in order to demonstrate that it is possible and reasonable for a person to stand up for himself. However, if he fights back too readily against unimportant accusations, he will leave the impression that he is weak or defensive, and thus that he has been hurt by the patient's criticisms. Also, if a therapist responds to the patient's tests in a stereotyped way, the patient may infer that the therapist is putting little effort into his work. The patient may then assume that the therapist is behaving in accordance with some preconceived technical prescriptions or rules.

FAILING THE PATIENT'S TESTS

Inevitably, the therapist fails some of the patient's tests or series of tests. When the failure is minor, the mistake may be corrected easily, and the therapist may learn from it. When the failure is major, it may be difficult to correct, and sometimes it cannot be corrected. In this section I discuss how the therapist may recognize when he has failed a test or a series of tests, how he may correct a minor failure after recognizing it, and how he may avoid serious failures.

Often the therapist may infer from the patient's response that he has failed a test. The patient usually reacts differently when the therapist fails a test than when he passes it. If the therapist fails a test by giving a poor intervention, the patient may respond less enthusiastically then usual, or he may become slightly depressed or silent. Also, he may fail to bring forth new material, or he may ignore the interpretation or change the topic. If the patient responds in one of these ways, the therapist may ask him, "How do you feel about what I just said?" or "Have I missed the point of what you were saying?"

Once the therapist begins to understand how he has failed a particular test, he may explain his failure to the patient. For example, he may tell a patient, "When you were complaining, you wanted me to help you realize you had a right to complain. Therefore, you were disappointed when I tried to encourage you. You took this to mean that I didn't want to hear your complaints."

After Failing a Minor Test

Sometimes after he fails a minor test, the therapist may simply wait for the patient to offer him a new chance by giving him another test similar to the one he failed. For example, a patient was burdened by the belief that he could force authorities to give him whatever he wanted. He provocatively demanded an extra hour and became upset when the therapist granted his request. The therapist realized he had made a mistake, but rather than pointing this out, he waited for the patient to test him again. A few sessions later, the patient asked to be permitted to miss several sessions without being charged, and he was relieved when the therapist refused him.

Sometimes after the therapist fails a test, the patient will coach him on how to pass it. The therapist in most instances should heed the patient's coaching. This may be illustrated by the example of a patient who suffered from the belief that if he criticized the therapist he would upset him. He tested this belief by criticizing the therapist, telling him, "I appreciate your readiness to be helpful. However, I'm hurt that you don't think I can solve problems myself. You don't seem to value my opinions and judgment." The therapist tried to reassure the patient by telling him that he did respect and appreciate his abilities and judgment. However, the patient felt not reassured but disappointed. He assumed that the therapist was being defensive and thus that he had hurt him. Therefore, before giving him a new test, he told the therapist how much his girlfriend was benefiting from the way her therapist dealt with her complaints. His girlfriend's therapist would simply point out how uncomfortable she (the girlfriend) felt when complaining about the therapist. The next time the patient complained, the therapist pointed out his discomfort with complaining. The patient appreciated the therapist's change of approach and elaborated on his fear of hurting the therapist.

Sometimes the patient signals the therapist that he is failing a test or a series of tests by ignoring the therapist's incorrect responses to his testing. This has been illustrated above in the analysis of Felice M., who ignored the analyst's offer to reduce her sessions from four to three times a week. It is also illustrated in the analysis of Lyle K., presented below.

Lyle K.

Lyle K., a successful lawyer, had felt rejected by both parents in childhood. In his analysis he began giving the therapist rejection tests several months after starting treatment, and continued to give him such tests every 2 or 3 months. The patient would tell the analyst that he had achieved his purposes, then complain about the cost of the treatment and state that he wanted to terminate. The analyst would challenge the patient's wish to stop, point to the patient's progress, and indicate that the patient had more to accomplish. The patient would react by briefly continuing to assert his wish to stop; he would then seem relieved and would agree to continue. Lyle made steady progress, and after $5\frac{1}{2}$ years of treatment the analyst began to assume that the patient might in fact be ready to terminate. Therefore, the next time Lyle threatened to stop, the analyst—unaware that he was being given the same kind of test as before—began seriously to explore the possibility of stopping. Lyle became slightly depressed and changed the subject. He discontinued his threats to stop for fear that the analyst would permit him to stop. He did not mention the possibility of stopping for the next 8 months, and then offered such weak arguments for stopping that he made the analyst aware that he did not wish to stop.

Sometimes the therapist may infer that he has failed an important test if the therapy becomes stalemated, as when, for example, a patient who is usually talkative becomes relatively silent for several weeks. If this happens, the therapist should try to remember when the stalemate began. He should also discuss it with the patient and should ask him how he thinks it started. An example of the development and resolution of a stalemate is presented below.

Donald G.

In his childhood Donald G. experienced his parents as weak and fragile. He suffered from the belief that he could make his parents obey him, and in order to protect them he kept himself indecisive. After $4\frac{1}{2}$ years of analysis, in which he made considerable progress, he began to test his belief in his omnipotence by criticizing the analyst. On one occasion, after criticizing the analyst, Donald angrily demanded to know when the analyst would consider the analysis finished. The analyst did not believe that the patient was ready to terminate. However, instead of simply stating this, the analyst, who was intimidated by the patient's angry criticisms, told him that he might be able to finish in a year. The patient seemed pleased by this possibility.

A few days afterwards, the analyst went away for summer

vacation. When Donald resumed therapy in the fall, he was uncharacteristically silent, and despite the analyst's attempts to understand this he remained silent. He continued to be silent for about a month until the analyst conjectured that the patient was upset about the termination plans. He asked the patient whether he had felt angry or rejected. Donald acknowledged that he felt these ways. Then he added that he feared he had forced the analyst to agree to his termination before the analyst believed he was ready. After this, the patient began to talk freely and to bring out new material.

Sometimes the therapist fails a test early in the therapy, before he understands his patient, but does not realize this until the patient tells him about it much later. This recurred in the analysis of a young woman who, late in treatment, reported the following episode: "I had been in analysis several weeks, and I came into your office about 3 minutes before you. I saw a small copper ashtray on your desk. I was tempted to steal it by slipping it into my handbag. I actually put it in the bag, but then took it out again and put it back on the desk. I began my hour that day by telling you about this temptation, and you said little about it. I got depressed. I wanted you to realize that I had a problem." The patient, in explaining why she had been disappointed with the therapist, pointed out that both of her parents were "Pollyannas" who were unable to criticize or confront her. When the therapist ignored the patient's worry that she might steal the ashtray, the patient feared that the therapist was like her Pollyanna parents, and so would be unable to help her.

After Failing a Major Test

The failure of a test or a series of tests is damaging if the patient reacts by giving up an important unconscious goal. It is especially damaging if the patient gives the therapist no indication that he is giving up the goal. It may be devastating if the patient, in obedience to his pathogenic beliefs, feels obliged to make a self-destructive decision that he cannot easily correct.

Below, I first present two cases in which a therapist's failures resulted in the patient's making a self-destructive decision. Then I discuss how such failures may be prevented.

Davis F.

A patient, Davis F., came to therapy with the goal of breaking up with a woman he had been going with for about 2 years. He sought support against his belief that since she was so attached to him, he had no right to leave her. The patient tested the therapist's willingness to help him leave the girlfriend by reporting that he now realized he was obligated to her, for during the time he was going with her she could have met other men. The therapist did not react to the patient's comments, and the patient took his silence as agreement. The patient, as a consequence of the therapist's failure to pass this test and a number of similar ones, felt compelled to marry the woman. The therapist failed this test, but never realized his failure. The patient reported this episode in his next therapy— an analysis he undertook for marital problems.

In the next example, the therapist's failure to pass a particular kind of test was devastating to the patient.

Allan C.

The patient, Allan C., a male social worker, suffered from the belief that he was a disgusting person who was hurtful to others and deserving of rejection. After 3 years of analysis, Allan tested this belief with the analyst by telling him that he wasn't making progress in therapy and wished to quit. The analyst readily agreed and set a termination date for 3 weeks from that date.

Allan felt terrible. He inferred from the analyst's willingness to let him go that either the analyst felt hurt and rejected, or he considered the patient worthless and untreatable. The patient was so upset that he quit his job and moved to another city, where he took up residence in a commune. After about a year, he pulled himself together and started treatment with another analyst. The story of his rejection by the first analyst did not come to light until after he had seen the second analyst for several years and had repeatedly tested the second analyst by criticizing him for his behavior as an analyst. The fact that the second analyst took the patient's criticisms seriously, and was neither hurt by them nor tempted to react to them by rejecting the patient, enabled the patient to remember how he assumed he had hurt the previous analyst.

How to Avoid Failing Important Tests

In order to minimize the chances of making serious errors, the therapist should keep in mind the best hypothesis he can make about the patient's pathogenic beliefs, goals, and plans. The therapist who failed to intervene when Davis F. stated how obligated he felt to his girlfriend was unaware that the patient was suffering from a powerful unconscious belief in his omnipotent responsibility for women; the therapist who took Allan C.'s wish to stop treatment at face value was unaware of the patient's fear of hurting him and sensitivity to rejection by him.

If the therapist who is being tested by the patient's indecisiveness is not sure what the patient really wants to do, he may discuss this with the patient. He may say, "I think you should delay this decision until you're sure of it." Or he may ask a patient who is considering taking an important initiative, "How would you feel if I encouraged you, or if I did not encourage you?" If the therapist is concerned that a patient in making a decision is motivated by a wish to placate him, the therapist may tell the patient, "Whatever you decide here is fine with me. But you should take your time, so as to be sure the decision is the one you really want to make."

If the therapist is unsure about the motives underlying the patient's wish to stop treatment, he should generally urge the patient to take his time about deciding. The therapist's urging the patient to postpone the decision will generally do little harm. However, the therapist, in not urging delay, may fail a rejection test. This may result in serious harm that cannot easily be repaired.

The therapist should always be aware that the patient in making a decision may be motivated by an unconscious wish to comply with him. Unconscious compliance to authority is universal. During the first few years of life every child regards his parents as absolute authorities. Some patients, especially at the beginning of treatment, may be so compliant that the therapist is impeded in his treatment of them. With such a patient the therapist is deprived of feedback, and therefore he may have difficulty in inferring the patient's plans; he may not know whether he is passing or failing the patient's tests. The therapist treating such a patient should be especially careful not to impose his own ideas on the patient inadvertently, and not to take the patient's agreeing with him as evidence that he is on the right track.

In most instances the highly compliant patient has the goal of overcoming his compliance, but cannot make this goal evident for fear of hurting the therapist. However, the highly compliant patient may be responsive to the therapist's attempts to help him overcome his compliance. In some instances the therapist should discuss the problem with the patient, being careful in doing so to avoid giving the impression that he is criticizing the patient or expecting a quick resolution of the problem. The therapist should attempt to find out the nature of the pathogenic beliefs underlying the patient's compliance. Many extremely compliant patients are burdened unconsciously with an intense sense of omnipotent responsibility for others. Such a patient may be afraid to express his opinions for fear of hurting the therapist and risking punishment and rejection from him. Perhaps he experienced his parents as fragile and kept himself highly compliant to protect their sense of authority, or perhaps they were extremely intolerant of any disagreement.

It is hard to overestimate the importance of unconscious compliance in the mental life of most patients. The therapist should not expect a patient to give up such compliance easily; the patient may be unable to do this. However, the therapist should try to prevent the patient from letting his wish to please the therapist interfere with important decisions.

SUMMARY

Throughout therapy, the patient tests his pathogenic beliefs with the therapist in the hope of disproving them. In a sense the patient is always testing the therapist, since he is always attempting to infer whether the therapist will help him to disprove his pathogenic beliefs and to pursue his goals. However, most patients test their pathogenic beliefs especially vigorously at times, and they do this throughout therapy. During these times, they behave in a way especially calculated to give them more explicit knowledge of the therapist's attitude toward their pathogenic beliefs and goals. For example, a patient who fears rejection may offer the therapist a powerful rejection test by threatening to quit treatment, hoping that the therapist will urge him to continue.

Some testing behavior is indistinguishable from ordinary behavior; however, some tests have special characteristics. The therapist may assume that the patient is testing him if the patient arouses powerful affects in him, forces him to intervene, or behaves much more foolishly or self-destructively than usual.

A patient may test by transferring or by turning passive into active. When a patient tests by transferring, he repeats with the therapist behavior similar to the behavior that in childhood he experienced as provoking his parents to traumatize him. He hopes that the therapist will not react to him as his parents reacted. When the patient tests by turning passive into active, he repeats the parental behavior that traumatized him. He hopes that the therapist will not be traumatized as he was, and thus that the therapist will provide him with a model of how to deal with the behavior that he experienced as traumatizing.

The patient may test by turning passive into active before taking an initiative that he considers dangerous. Through such testing he confronts the therapist with the dangers that he anticipates, hoping that the therapist will provide him with a model for dealing successfully with such dangers.

If the therapist feels extremely upset, worried, humiliated, or uncomfortable with the patient, the patient is almost always turning passive into active. He is repeating parental behavior that he experienced as extremely distressing. The reason why transference tests are generally much easier for the therapist to tolerate than passive-into-active tests is evident from the lopsided relationship of children to parents. A child is highly motivated to get along with his parents and will rarely do anything to greatly disturb a parent. However, a parent may not be highly motivated to get along with a child; a parent may worry a child, reject him, beat him, or abandon him.

A patient may test the therapist by proposing a course of

action that he assumes the therapist wants him to take, but that from the therapist's point of view is self-destructive. Therefore, the therapist should be especially careful to give the patient an opportunity to reverse a decision that may be against the patient's interests. The therapist should make clear to the patient that he may take as much time as he needs to make the decision, and that the therapist will support any reasonable decision that the patient makes.

CHAPTER 6

INTERPRETATION

The therapist may use interpretations for a variety of purposes. He may use them to pass the patient's tests, to help the patient feel more secure in therapy, and to help the patient see himself more sympathetically. Also, the therapist may use interpretations to help the patient become conscious of his pathogenic beliefs and goals, and thus to work more effectively at disproving these beliefs and pursuing these goals.

Interpretations may provide the patient with explanations (Bibring, 1954) that help him to understand his development and his psychopathology. For example, he may learn that he developed maladaptive beliefs in his attempts to maintain his ties to his parents, and that these beliefs require him, for example, to maintain his psychopathology out of loyalty to his parents. Such explanations may be demystifying and normalizing. They may help the patient to realize that he is not inherently bad, perverse, crazy, or borderline, and that the symptoms that make him ashamed and guilty are readily understood in terms of his childhood experiences and his attempts to cope with them.

The value of the therapist's interpretations depends not simply on the knowledge they convey, but on the authority of the therapist who conveys this knowledge. A patient may have considerable understanding of his psychopathology, yet be unable to use this self-knowledge constructively. However, the same knowledge conveyed by the therapist may be quite helpful. For example, a patient may know that he is not protecting himself from certain dangers, but be unable to give himself the protection he needs. However, he may be helped if told by his therapist that he deserves to be protected, especially if he becomes convinced that the therapist wants him to avoid taking unnecessary risks. In this case, as in all instances of the successful use of interpretation, the patient relies on the therapist's authority to help him do what he unconsciously wants to do. It is one thing for a patient to know that he wants to go in a certain direction; it is another thing for him to realize that a person whom he endows with considerable authority wants him to go in that direction and will help him to do so.

THE THERAPIST'S FIRST PRIORITY: HELPING THE PATIENT FEEL SAFE

The therapist's concern for helping the patient to feel safe takes precedence over his attempts to give the patient insight by interpretation. In those instances in which the patient is threatened by any interpretation, the therapist should refrain from interpreting until the patient can safely tolerate his doing so. This applies to the patient who likens the therapist's interpretations to his parents' lecturing him, pulling rank, or giving unsolicited advice.

If the therapist succeeds by noninterpretative means in providing the patient with a sense of safety, the patient may begin to develop insights on his own. He may remember more about his childhood traumas and become more aware of his pathogenic beliefs and goals. At this point, the therapist may add to the patient's developing self-knowledge by providing explanations that the patient can use to organize this knowledge and to fit it into a comprehensive picture of his personality and development. This may be illustrated by the example of Thomas C. (see Chapter 4).

Thomas E. (Continued)

As noted in Chapter 4, Thomas C.'s parents were critical, allowed him little or no freedom, and insisted that he work most of the time. At the beginning of treatment, almost any interpretation made the patient feel uncomfortable. He would experience an interpretation as an infringement on his freedom. He wanted unconsciously to feel free with the therapist and to be accepted by him, and the therapist tried to help him to feel these ways by treating him noninterpretatively. The therapist chatted informally with Thomas about almost any topic that Thomas introduced.

After only several weeks of therapy, the patient began to feel safe enough to produce new memories and insights. After a number of months, the patient was talking easily about how he valued a sense of freedom and how he felt confined by even a loose schedule. He also linked his need for freedom to the constraints his parents had imposed on him. At this point, the therapist demonstrated sympathy with the patient's striving for freedom and offered the patient a conceptual framework for understanding how he came to feel constrained. The therapist pointed out that the patient had complied with his parents' restrictions. He had come to believe that his parents were right to restrict him, and thus that he was not supposed to feel free.

As a consequence of these and other comments, the patient became less averse to interpretation. Though the therapist continued to treat the patient mainly by his attitude, he made a number of comments designed to help the patient to fit his memories and ideas into a broad explanatory framework, thereby helping the patient to understand himself better and to see himself more sympathetically.

CHARACTERISTICS OF GOOD INTERPRETATIONS

Good Interpretations Are Not Neutral

The patient is always in psychic conflict. He wants to work at disproving his pathogenic beliefs and pursuing his goals, but in order to do this, he must defy his pathogenic beliefs and thus experience anxiety. In this conflict the therapist is never neutral. He is always on the side of the patient's attempts to solve his problems. Moreover, even if the therapist tries to be neutral, the patient does not experience him this way. The patient relates everything the therapist says to his efforts to disprove his pathogenic beliefs; therefore, he experiences the therapist's comments either as sympathetic to his goals, as opposed to them, or as irrelevant to them.

Sometimes an interpretation may be true but anti-plan because it sends the wrong message to the patient. In such instances, the addition of a new element may make the interpretation compatible with the patient's plan. This may be illustrated by comparing the interpretation "You are critical of me" with the interpretation "You are uncomfortable about being critical of me." If the second interpretation is true, so is the first. Yet the two interpretations may carry quite different messages. The first interpretation implies that the patient should become aware that he is being critical and should stop being that way; the second implies that he should become aware that he is uncomfortable about being critical and should permit himself to be critical.

Whether one of these interpretations helps or hinders a particular patient or seems irrelevant to him depends on the nature of the patient's plan. If the patient is attempting to overcome his fear of criticizing others lest he hurt them, he may experience the interpretation "You are being critical" as a complaint, and so may assume that he has hurt the therapist. If so, he may experience the interpretation as confirming his pathogenic belief. On the other hand, he may experience the comment "You are uncomfortable about being critical" as helping him to disprove the pathogenic belief, for he may assume from it that he has not hurt the therapist by criticizing him.

However, if the patient is struggling to face the fact of his aggression, he may find the interpretation "You are being critical" to be pro-plan. This was the case in the therapy of a patient whose Pollyanna parents failed to confront the patient's aggression. They never spoke about it and appeared not to notice it. The patient had inferred from this that his aggressive behavior was so unacceptable that it could not be talked about. The patient was therefore relieved at the therapist's blunt reference to his being critical.

The point that two interpretations, although both true, may carry different messages may also be illustrated by comparing the following interpretations: "You feel guilty about wanting to be independent of your parents" and "You are uncomfortable about being dependent on your parents." If the first interpretation is true, so is the second. Yet a patient may react quite differently to them. A patient who unconsciously is working to overcome separation guilt may be helped if told that he feels guilty about wanting to be more independent of his parents. However, he may be set back if told he is uncomfortable about depending on them, for he may experience this interpretation as telling him he should not try to be more independent.

In contrast, a patient who suffers from his fear of burdening others by needing them may benefit from an interpretation about his fear of dependency. This was the case in the therapy of a patient who wanted to rely on the therapist, but was afraid that the therapist would be burdened by his dependency. The patient was relieved when the therapist told him, "You are afraid of relying on me." The patient took the therapist's comment as evidence that the therapist would not feel drained by the patient's depending on him.

Good Interpretations Give the Patient Something He Wants to Receive

An interpretation is rarely helpful (pro-plan) unless it gives the patient something he unconsciously wants to receive. A good interpretation usually reduces the patient's level of anxiety, guilt, or shame. It may answer a question the patient is unconsciously asking. It may provide the patient with greater perspective on the course of his life or on the nature of his difficulties. It may help him to understand and forgive himself for behavior about which he feels ashamed or guilty. It may help him in his struggle to disprove a pathogenic belief. Unless the patient unconsciously wants to accept an interpretation, the interpretation will not be useful. If the interpretation is anti-plan, the patient will either ignore it, in which case it is ineffective, or comply with it, in which case it may be harmful.

The therapist cannot always assess the value (planfulness) of an interpretation by noting the patient's conscious reactions to it. A patient may consciously resist an interpretation that he unconsciously wants to accept; in doing this, he may hope to demonstrate to himself that the therapist has the courage of his convictions and so will stick with it.

This may be illustrated by the example of a patient who consciously resisted the therapist's efforts to show the patient that he was behaving provocatively. The patient was unconsciously identifying with his parents who characteristically denied their mistreatment of him. The patient would insult the therapist, misquote him, or underpay him, then deny that he had done such a thing. The patient was giving the therapist passive-into-active tests. He wanted the therapist to challenge his denials and to persist in challenging them despite his protests, so that he (the patient) could learn from the therapist how to challenge his parents' denials and to persist in challenging them.

In another case, too, a patient consciously resisted the therapist's efforts to confront him with his denials. However, he unconsciously welcomed the confrontations. The patient's parents had been unable to face their problems. They denied their poverty; they borrowed large sums of money and spent it as though they were rich. Also, the patient's father denied the severity of his chronic bronchitis: Though it was life-threatening he refused to go to a doctor. The patient unconsciously wanted to face his problems, but believed that by doing so he would be disloyal to his parents. He resisted the therapist's efforts to confront him with his poor management of his finances and his failure to take care of himself. However, he was unconsciously relieved when the therapist persisted, and over a period of time he benefited.

The Therapist Should Help the Patient Develop a Broad Perspective

The patient has a strong wish to develop a broad, coherent picture of his psychopathology and development, for such a picture helps him to see himself sympathetically and to increase his mastery over his problems and his personality. The therapist should help the patient to acquire such a picture. The therapist should help the patient to understand where he came from, where he wants to go, and how he plans to get there. Once the therapist has helped the patient develop a broad picture of himself, the therapist should try to relate the patient's new productions to this picture, thereby changing the picture, adding to it, or filling in its details.

The more the therapist succeeds in putting the patient's productions into a broad perspective, the more he is likely to help him. Sometimes the patient is helped by simple comments, such as "You like to look," "You are hostile," "You are angry or dependent," or "You are withdrawn." More often, he is not. He may experience such comments as criticisms, because hostility, dependency, or withdrawal is generally not highly regarded. Nor do such comments help the patient to understand why he developed such motives or defenses; therefore, they may fail to help him to perceive himself sympathetically. A patient may want to know, "How did I become so interested in looking?" Other patients may want to know, "Why am I so dependent?" "Am I different from other people, and, if so, how did I get that way?" "Should I not be interested in looking?" "Should I stop being dependent, and, if so, how do I go about doing so?"

Any perspective that the therapist adds to a simple statement of the patient's impulses or defenses may be helpful. Thus it may be helpful if the therapist shows the patient that his behavior was developed to serve some reasonable unconscious moral or adaptive purpose (e.g., to express loyalty to parents, to make amends for being better off than siblings, or to adapt to an interpersonal world he perceived as hostile or unrewarding). Such explanations make intuitive sense. They help the patient to see himself sympathetically, and to feel normal and good as opposed to abnormal and bad. They help the patient forgive himself for behavior he considers shameful or reprehensible.

The treatment of the seemingly intractable patient described in Chapter 5, who tests the therapist by turning passive into active, illustrates the value of showing the patient through interpretation that his behavior has an adaptive function or serves an unconscious moral purpose. Such interpretation may help the seemingly impossible patient to understand his behavior; to feel less guilty about it; and to relate it to his childhood experiences, his pathogenic beliefs, and his goals. Thus a seemingly impossible patient may be helped if told that he is being difficult out of loyalty to parents whom he experienced as impossible (and thus that his behavior serves a moral purpose); or that he is being difficult to show the therapist how he felt in childhood with an impossible parent (and thus that his behavior serves the purpose of advancing the therapy); or that he is being difficult to test the therapist (and thus that he is working to change a pathogenic belief).

The Patient May Benefit from Interpretations That Help Him to Develop the Strength to Protect Himself

A patient may be unable to develop close relations with others because he lacks the capacity to protect himself from the danger that he assumes is inherent in close relationships. If so, his plan may require him to work in therapy, sometimes for long periods of time, to develop the capacity to protect himself from the perceived danger. The therapist may use interpretation to help the patient to develop this capacity. Then, after the patient has accomplished this, he may permit himself the close relationships that he feared earlier.

Consider, for example, a male patient who was unable to say "no" to his girlfriend. He was afraid to fall in love with her for fear that he would have to comply with all her wishes. He worked to develop the capacity to say "no" to her, and was helped to acquire this capacity when the therapist pointed out his fear of refusing her, lest he hurt her. After the patient was able to say "no" to her, he permitted himself to feel close to her.

Another example concerns a patient who, when shamed by another person, felt compelled to comply by feeling ashamed. This patient was so afraid of being shamed that he was unable to feel comfortable with others. He was helped when the therapist made him aware of his belief that he would hurt a person if he did not comply with that person's wish to shame him. As he became able to resist being shamed, he became more comfortable in social relations.

If a patient appears to make difficulties for himself by being stubborn, the therapist may err if he attempts to make the patient aware of his stubbornness with the implied purpose of inducing him to stop being stubborn. In some instances, depending on the patient's plan, the therapist should do the opposite. The patient may be testing him by a show of stubbornness as part of his working to acquire the right to be stubborn. If so, the patient's stubbornness is counterphobic. Although he may seem comfortable being stubborn, he is unconsciously anxious or guilty about being that way. The therapist may then be most helpful by interpreting the patient's unconscious guilt about his stubbornness, thereby helping him acquire the ability to avoid self-destructive compliance. As he develops the capacity not to comply with others, he may permit himself to feel close to them. Paradoxically, then, the therapist, by helping the patient to acquire the capacity to resist the demands of others, may enable him to get along better with them.

It is often futile to tell a patient who is bragging that he is feeling proud in order to ward off his sense of humiliation. The patient may experience the therapist who does this as wanting to put him down, and so as repeating a parental mistake. On the other hand, if the therapist points out the patient's unconscious fear or guilt about feeling proud, the patient may develop the self-esteem necessary to acknowledge his shortcomings. In addition, he may feel less compelled to brag.

The same applies to the patient whose tendency to blame others appears to be an obstacle to his feeling close to them. Here too, depending on the patient's unconscious plan, the therapist may err if he attempts to induce the patient to stop blaming others by interpreting his tendency to blame them. The patient who blames others may unconsciously be vulnerable to being blamed, and so may believe that any criticisms he receives are deserved. He may blame others to protect himself from feeling blamed. In this case, the patient, if told by the therapist that he is blaming others to protect himself from guilt, may simply feel blamed. He may assume that the therapist wants him to feel guilt. He may then feel endangered by the therapist and fight back by blaming him.

In treating a patient with this kind of problem, the therapist may help the patient by showing him that he is too ready to accept blame from others, and that unconsciously he has difficulty knowing when others are in fact blaming him unfairly. If the patient is helped to stop complying with unfair blame, and to know when others are treating him unfairly, he may become less vulnerable to them and have less need to protect himself from guilt by blaming them.

This point is illustrated by the patient mentioned in Chapter 2 who repeatedly blamed his mother for her mistreatment of him. This patient continued to blame her until the therapist agreed that she had mistreated him, and that the patient had blamed himself unfairly for her abusive behavior. The patient became relieved. In addition, he acknowledged that on a few occasions he had provoked his mother.

There are always exceptions to the principles presented above. Though often a patient is set back when told that he is stubborn, vainglorious, or blaming, he may in some instances benefit. For example, the patient may be maintaining his unfavorable behavior in order to punish himself, perhaps out of compliance to a parent to whom he feels guilty. The patient may unconsciously be highly motivated to give up the unfavorable behavior, but may believe that he should not. In such instances the therapist's direct attempts to make the patient aware of his unfavorable behavior, with the implication that he should give it up, may be helpful. This reminds us again that the only technical rule broad enough to include most instances is that the therapist should help the patient to carry out his unconscious plan.

Interpretations May Be Helpful if They Imply a Promise Not to Mistreat the Patient

Sometimes the therapist may help the patient by pointing out the patient's irrational transference expectations. The therapist may do this by telling the patient, for example, "You're afraid that if you continue to attack me I will reject you," or "You're afraid that if you're proud I will put you down," or "You're afraid that if you're seductive I'll try to have sex with you," and so forth. Such interpretations may provide the patient with a sense of safety, for they imply a promise not to behave as the patient fears. It would be almost unthinkable for a therapist to imply by interpretation that he will not react as the patient fears, but then, having lulled the patient to feel secure, to go back on his implied promise.

This may be illustrated by the therapy of a young attorney who in childhood inferred from certain experiences with his father that if he were arrogant with an authority he would provoke ridicule. During the first few months of his therapy, the patient became anxious about expressing pride in his achievements and found relief when the therapist told him, "You are anxious because you are proud and are afraid that I'll ridicule you for your pride, as your father did." The patient was relieved by the interpretation, because he unconsciously inferred from it that the analyst would not ridicule him for his pride. He assumed that the analyst, after inducing him to display his pride, would not betray him by punishing him for it. As evidence that he felt relieved, he retrieved a new memory: When he was a young child, he would provoke his father by saying "I know" to everything his father told him.

Another patient, a young man, had indulged surreptitiously in sex play with his mother from early childhood until he was 13. He and his mother occasionally slept in the same bed, and while pretending to be asleep they would rub against each other. Neither the patient nor his mother ever alluded to this; the patient was not even sure that his mother had been aware of it. At one point in his therapy, the patient, despite his female therapist's correct, nonseductive demeanor, became unconsciously afraid that he would seduce her. However, he was relieved when the therapist told him, "You are afraid that you will seduce me as you believe you seduced your mother." The patient was helped by this interpretation to become aware of his fear of seducing the therapist, and to remember more about his sex play with his mother.

The patient gained relief from this interpretation because he inferred a promise from it. He took the analyst's discussing his fear that he would seduce her as a promise that she would not be seduced. He was reassured by the very fact that the analyst spoke openly about this fear. In his childhood he and his mother could continue their sex play, because by not talking about it they were not facing it.

ANTI-PLAN INTERPRETATIONS

If the therapist consistently makes anti-plan interpretations, the patient may fail to improve or, in some cases, he may stop treatment. This point may be illustrated by the case of Esther A.

Esther A.

In her childhood, Esther A. had felt cheated by her mother, whom she described as self-important and "queenly." According to Esther, her mother sometimes failed to keep her promises. She readily became impatient and screamed at the patient upon slight provocation, and she refused to listen to Esther's attempts to make herself understood.

Esther's conflict with her female therapist was confined to a particular situation. The therapist would be 1 or 2 minutes late for her appointment, but would not extend the session to make up for the lost time. Esther would complain provocatively that the therapist was irresponsible, cheated her, cut corners, failed to take her seriously, and so forth. The therapist would tell the patient that she was suffering from a mother transference, and so she felt cheated even though the therapist had no intention of cheating her. The therapist would explain that the occasional loss of a minute was inevitable and of no great importance, and that Esther was losing much more than a minute of her time by making such a fuss about it. If the patient had not felt cheated by her mother, she would scarcely have noticed the loss of a minute.

Esther was provoked rather than placated by such explanations. She insisted that the therapist was rationalizing her own irresponsible behavior. She acknowledged that she had felt cheated by her mother, but emphasized that this made the therapist's cheating her even less acceptable. The argument between therapist and patient went on throughout Esther's first therapy, which lasted for about a year. Sometimes the therapist would say, "Look, I'm not your mother," or "Can't you see that you were mad at your mother and now you're taking it out on me?" As a consequence of the therapist's adherence to her position, Esther decided to stop treatment, despite the fact that the therapist had been helpful.

A few months after stopping treatment with this therapist, Esther entered an analysis with another female therapist. She soon began to behave with the new analyst as she had with her first therapist. She would complain provocatively when the analyst came a minute late. However, the analyst reacted by agreeing with the patient. She would apologize for being late and agree to make up the time; she would then focus on Esther's discomfort with complaining about her behavior. She thereby helped the patient to realize that unconsciously she had felt guilty about her complaining.

The analyst emphasized that Esther had every right to complain. She pointed out that even though she was only a minute late, her being late carried a powerful symbolic meaning to the patient, for it confirmed her belief that she had no right to be treated fairly. Esther found the analyst's approach helpful. She came to understand that she had been concerned about being cheated because she had complied with her mother's cheating her, and so assumed that she deserved to be cheated. In her analysis, she was struggling to convince herself that she did not deserve this.

In the following example, the therapist persisted for some time in maintaining a certain plan formulation. He then found his mistake and, to the patient's benefit, corrected it.

Katherine A.

Katherine A., an intelligent woman of 30, had trouble keeping up with her monthly analytic fees. She complained to her analyst, at first mildly and then progressively more vituperatively, about his refusal to stretch out her payments. She screamed and sobbed at the analyst while criticizing him for his rigidity. She compared him to her stepfather, the only other person with whom the patient had ever lost her temper.

Katherine in early childhood had loved her father a great deal. She had been closer to him than to her mother, whom she considered both fragile and unattractive. Her parents, who were unhappily married, obtained a divorce when the patient was 8. She did not appear deeply upset about this, but was quite upset when during her 12th year her mother remarried. She took an immediate dislike to her stepfather, whom she considered an autocrat. She fought with him constantly.

The analyst assumed that the patient had been fighting with him about her payments because she had developed a stepfather transference. He attempted to deal with this transference both by interpreting it and by demonstrating in his behavior that he was not autocratic. Therefore he told the patient that he would allow her to delay her current payments by 1 month.

Katherine at first seemed overjoyed at the analyst's flexibility. However, she soon became even more discouraged and angry. The analyst, who now began to realize he was on the wrong track, consulted a colleague, who tentatively offered the following explanation for the patient's behavior:

Katherine had blamed herself in childhood for her parents' divorce. She assumed that her father found her so much more attractive than her mother that he stopped caring for her mother. After her mother remarried, the patient was determined to avoid repeating what she perceived as her Oedipal crime. She fought violently with her stepfather in order to make sure she was unattractive to him. In her current life, Katherine feared that she would seduce the analyst as she believed she had seduced her father; she fought with him, as she had fought with her stepfather, in order to make herself unattractive to him. The analyst's telling her that she would be allowed to defer her current payment was frightening, for the patient inferred from it that she was indeed seducing the analyst.

Several months after his meeting with the consultant, the analyst had a good opportunity to check this formulation. The patient reported that she had begun to worry about her relations with her boyfriend. She was not sure she loved him; in fact, she had a strong suspicion that she was involved with him for some neurotic reason. The analyst assumed that Katherine was describing doubt about her love for her boyfriend in order to determine whether the analyst, out of envy, would agree with her doubts. He told her "It seems to me from what you've said about your boyfriend that you do love him, and that you are reluctant to say so for fear I will feel left out." This time Katherine reacted favorably to the analyst's comments. After this, she became encouraged and by her associations confirmed his point. She became more friendly to the analyst and less concerned about his rigidity.

TRANSFERENCE INTERPRETATIONS VERSUS NONTRANSFERENCE INTERPRETATIONS

The importance of transference interpretations is exaggerated by certain contemporary authors.[1] A research study[2] carried out by Polly Fretter (Silberschatz, Fretter, & Curtis, 1986) showed that transference interpretations are no more and no less beneficial than nontransference interpretations. The important distinction is not between transference and nontrans-

---

[1]For a similar assessment, see Rangell (1981a) and Lomas (1982).

[2]This study was carried out under the supervision of Curtis and Silberschatz.

ference interpretations, but between pro-plan and anti-plan interpretations.

Also, the therapist may pass a patient's transference tests without referring explicitly to the patient's relationship with him. Consider, for example, a patient who is afraid to report an achievement for fear the therapist will belittle him. The patient may benefit from the therapist's making a transference interpretation, such as "You're afraid to tell me about your success for fear I will belittle it." However, the patient may benefit just as much if the therapist responds to the patient's reporting his success by saying, "That's good news." In both instances the patient will realize that the therapist is not motivated to belittle him. Just which approach is better for a particular patient depends on many factors. The patient who wants the therapist to be careful, deliberate, and analytic may prefer the former approach. The patient who feels put down by interpretation may prefer the latter.

CHAPTER 7

The Therapist's Use of Dreams

DREAMS AND THEIR ADAPTIVE FUNCTIONS

What can the patient and the therapist learn from the patient's dreams? How may the therapist use what he learns to help the patient? In this chapter I propose a theory of dreams intended to throw light on these questions. This theory is consistent with the assumptions about the mind and motivation presented in Chapter 1. It assumes that a person, in his dreams as in his conscious waking life, thinks about his reality and attempts to adapt to it.[1] A person's dreams are products of normal (albeit unconscious), thoughts, and they express his attempts at adaptation. He produces dreams in an effort to deal with current concerns that he has not resolved by waking thoughts, either because these concerns are too overwhelming, because he is hampered in his thinking about them by his pathogenic beliefs, or because he has not had time to think about them. A person may sometimes reveal more self-knowledge and may see things more clearly in his dreams than in his waking life.

In his dreams a person may assess situations and develop plans for dealing with them much as he does in waking life. He may alert himself to a problem that he has overlooked, make a resolution, remind himself of a new insight, console himself for a loss, or reprimand himself for a misdeed. He may prepare for

[1]For empirical evidence that dreams are adaptive, see Winson (1990) and Greenberg, Katz, Schwartz, and Pearlman (1992).

an upcoming task by encouraging himself; or he may bring forth repressed traumatic experiences so as to make himself aware of the traumas and to master the affects connected with them; or he may tell himself more clearly than in waking life how he feels about someone who is close to him; and so forth. In a sense a person, by producing a dream, sends a message to himself.

Though dreams are products of thoughts that are similar to waking thoughts, they nonetheless may appear mysterious to the dreamer. There are several reasons for this. The dream is an isolated production, for the dreamer while dreaming is unaware of the events and the thoughts about them that gave rise to the dream. Also, the dreamer may be unaware of his attitude to the dream. For example, he may not know during the dream that he is expressing his ideas through the use of irony or metaphor. In addition, since the dream is expressed in visual images, it cannot represent logical relations. For example, a person who fears that if he continues to be provocative he will be punished, may in a dream warn himself against the danger of punishment simply by depicting himself being punished. Finally, since the dream is not intended to communicate except to the dreamer, it may rely on highly idiosyncratic ideas, comparisons, or metaphors to express its meaning.

DREAMS OF PRISONERS OF WAR: EXAMPLES OF THE ADAPTIVE FUNCTIONS OF DREAMS

The adaptive functions of dreams may be illustrated by Balson's (1975) study of the dreams of five soldiers who had been prisoners of war in Vietnam.[2] According to Balson, these soldiers produced typical dreams in the following three situations:

1. When they were in danger of being captured.
2. During long imprisonment in which they were mistreated.
3. After their release from prison camp.

[2]For further discussion of these dreams, see Weiss et al. (1986), Chapter 7.

When in danger of capture, the soldiers typically produced frightening dreams of being captured. This kind of dream was a warning dream. In it the dreamers told themselves, "Be careful or this may happen." Dreams have no way of representing such conjunctions as "if" in pictorial form (Freud, 1900, p. 429). The best they could do in this case was to represent the possibility of capture by depicting the situation of capture.

The soldiers' warning dreams were adaptive. Such dreams oriented them throughout the night to the danger they were facing and thereby prepared them for it. The dreams performed this function whether or not they were interpreted or understood.[3] They kept the dreamers aware of the possibility of capture, and by preventing them from sleeping too soundly, they made them less vulnerable to capture.

During prolonged internment in which they were treated badly, the soldiers produced blissful dreams of gratification, power, and serenity. By producing these dreams, the soldiers helped themselves to adapt to their situation. They defied their tormentors and offered themselves a measure of hope. They also helped themselves sleep deeply, and thus restored themselves. These blissful dreams were important to the soldiers; they remembered them vividly long afterward, and during waking hours they would console themselves by dwelling on them.

In everyday life blissful dreams are rare. A person does not permit them, lest he lull himself into a false sense of security and so fail to prepare himself for the problems he must face upon awakening. However, a captured soldier was unable to affect his fate, and so had nothing to lose by denying his painful reality; his turning from reality in his dreams did not make his situation more dangerous.

After they were released from camp, the soldiers produced the kind of traumatic dreams that Freud discussed in *Beyond*

---

[3]For empirical evidence that certain kinds of dreams may perform their adaptive functions whether or not they are interpreted, see Greenberg et al. (1992).

the Pleasure Principle (1920). The purpose of these dreams, Freud argued, is not gratification but mastery. After their release, the soldiers felt safe, and so could begin the work of lifting their repressions and remembering the horrifying experiences of capture and internment. Their purpose in these dreams was to master the horror and fear connected with the traumatic experiences and to change the pathogenic beliefs inferred from them. In such dreams the soldiers were not simply planning to remember the traumatic experiences so as to master them; they were beginning to carry out this plan.

A DREAM MAY CARRY A SIMPLE
BUT IMPORTANT MESSAGE

As illustrated by the dreams of the prisoners of war studied by Balson, a dream may carry a relatively simple but important message to the dreamer. The soldiers who dreamed they were being captured told themselves, "Be careful, or you will be captured." The soldiers who in prison camp produced blissful dreams told themselves, "Have hope! You may again experience such pleasures." The soldiers who after release from prison camp began to remember their horrifying experiences there were setting forth a plan and beginning to carry it out: "Remember and master what you have suffered."

My emphasis on the simple but profound message that a dream conveys to the dreamer agrees with Freud's conclusions about a number of dreams in *The Interpretation of Dreams* (1900). The dream interpretations that Freud proposed there are all simple. They contain simple ideas, or several related ideas that are easily encompassed in one or two sentences by a more general statement. The impression of complexity that Freud conveyed in his analysis of certain of his own dreams is not in their meanings, but in the elaborate and intertwining associations that Freud produced in his efforts to arrive at their meanings. For example, Freud took over 10 pages to report his associations to the dream of Irma's injection (1900, pp. 106–120). However, according to his interpretation, this dream carried a simple but important message—namely, that he, Freud, was not responsible for not curing Irma.

Also, Freud wrote that examination dreams typically carry a simple but important message of encouragement (1900, pp. 273–276). They tell the dreamer that he need not worry about an upcoming task, for though he once worried that he would fail at a similar task, he in fact carried it out successfully.

Often the message that a dreamer is sending himself is not intelligible from the dream's imagery. In these instances, the interpreter may not understand the dream until the dreamer reveals his attitude to the dream imagery and thus suggests a caption for the dream. For example, a patient who dreams he is walking down a road by himself may be expressing a wish, a fear, or an expectation. He may be telling himself, "I hope I'll be in this situation," or "I'm afraid I'll be in this situation," or "If I finish my work, I'll be able to put myself in this situation," or "If I continue to provoke my colleagues, I'll find myself in this situation."

Sometimes the caption the dreamer intends may readily be inferred from the situation in which the dreamer produced the dream. This applies to the dreams of the soldiers who feared capture and who dreamed that they were being captured. It also applies to the dreams of the tormented prisoners who dreamed of power and serenity.

The idea that a caption may make a dream intelligible can be illustrated by the dream of a depressed patient who felt guilty complaining about his unhappy childhood. He dreamed he was having a happy Christmas with his family. The dream made sense when the dreamer, in commenting about the dream, supplied this caption: "Life was never like this."

HOW THE DREAMER GIVES THE DREAM MEANING

The dreamer may use a variety of techniques to create a dream that embodies his message to himself. Indeed, as will be seen, a dreamer in creating his dreams may use many of the techniques familiar to us from waking thought and from literature. He relies on the content and form of the dream to give it meaning.[4]

In his dreams he may tell a simple story realistically, as in the warning dreams and the blissful dreams of Balson's prisoners of war. He may rely on irony, as in the dream of the man who reminded himself of his unhappy childhood by depicting himself as a child enjoying Christmas with his family. He may, by a dream of utter confusion, warn himself that he faces a task that will require him to keep his wits about him so as to avoid confusion. He may convey his message by metaphor. His dream may have the characteristics of a sitcom, a farce, or a black comedy. Dreams may be light and witty, or they may carry the authority and solemnity of an Old Testament prophecy.

In a number of dreams that I have studied, the dreamer constructs a dream in the form of an argument, using the logical technique of "reduction to absurdity." He attempts to disprove a particular premise by showing that the premise leads to an absurd conclusion. The use of reduction to absurdity is common not only in dreams but in waking thought. It is normal in making a plan to deduce what will happen if the plan is carried out. If the consequences of carrying it out are absurd, then the plan is seen as flawed.

A dream reflecting the use of reduction to absurdity was produced by a young woman who, after beginning an affair, felt disloyal and guilty to her twin sister. She had assumed that she should be able to attain everything she wanted in her relationship with her sister. In the dream, she was married to her sister

---

[4]My view that both the content of the dream and its form may be central to its meaning contrasts with Freud's account as presented in his early works (1900, 1901, Vol. 4, pp. 118–121). In Freud's account, the story of the dream may be a product of secondary revision, which the dream work carries out on the dream contents in order to make the dream intelligible. Also, the dreamer may produce an utterly confusing dream if the dream work fails to make the dream contents intelligible. Thus in Freud's view neither the dream story nor the form of the dream is necessarily central to its meaning, but merely the result of the success or failure of the dream work in making the dream thoughts intelligible.

My approach to dreams is much more compatible with the ideas about dreams that Freud presented in his later works. For a brief history of Freud's theorizing and the theorizing of other analysts about dreams, see Weiss et al. (1986), Chapter 7.

and they were having a baby. By this dream, the dreamer reduced this assumption to absurdity, and justified her right to have the affair. The caption of the dream and of the thought to which it gave rise might be "This is absurd."

Examination dreams as described by Freud (1900) are in some ways similar to dreams that rely on reduction to absurdity. In examination dreams, the dreamer encourages himself by dreaming that he has failed a test that in fact he passed. His intention is to tell himself that his worries are absurd. In examination dreams, as in other dreams of reduction to absurdity, the dreamer does not express his confidence in himself directly. In my experience, patients who produce examination dreams are uncomfortable about feeling confident. In several such instances, the patient was unconsciously confident of himself; however, as a consequence of his survivor guilt toward his parents, he felt obliged to worry about upcoming tasks.

The examples offered below are not intended as evidence for my theory of dreams, but as illustrations of this theory and of its application to the treatment of patients. In my opinion, an investigator cannot provide convincing evidence for a dream theory except by use of formal research techniques, because in selecting his evidence he is inevitably guided by his basic ideas about the nature of dreams and their relation to mental functioning. Moreover, the examples presented below are of dreams that both the therapist and the patient understood or thought they understood relatively easily, perhaps after the patient had thought briefly about the dreams or offered a few associations to them. (Freud reported that dreams that are easily understood are quite common; "they wear their meanings on their faces" [1900, p. 126]).

Most dreams are not as readily understood as those reported here, in some instances because the metaphors or other devices the dreamer uses are quite idiosyncratic. Some dreams remain obscure, despite the patient's spending considerable effort in free-associating to the dreams and in thinking about their messages. However, even obscure dreams, once understood, can be seen to serve the same purposes and to use the same techniques as the dreams presented here.

The first example is of a dream that made its point by use

of reduction to absurdity. It occurred in the analysis of a young man.

> In this dream, which took place in the world of science fiction, a number of female creatures came to earth. They looked like the blue ice used in coolers. Two of them were attempting to seduce an earth man who was lying on his back. One was on each ankle. The dreamer, who observed this, thought, "This doesn't seem too exciting." This thought might serve as the dream's caption.

After the dreamer's first comment, which was about how unsatisfactory the blue ice females would be as sexual partners, he became clear about the dream's meaning. Without realizing it, he had been impeded in his sex life with his girlfriend by his irrational fear of contamination. The message in the dream was that, though in his opinion the human body was unclean, a perfectly clean pure sex object would be completely boring. He told himself that what he wanted was a warm human woman, even though he assumed she might not be completely clean. The dreamer gave himself his message indirectly, because he felt guilty about telling himself directly to ignore his squeamishness and enjoy sex with his girlfriend. He believed that to do this would be disloyal to his squeamish, timid mother.

In the next example, the patient used metaphor to tell himself something in his dream that he was not quite ready to acknowledge in his waking life.

> He dreamed that he and some friends were spending a pleasant afternoon near his family's summer cottage on a lake in Quebec. It was a beautiful day and they were taking a walk. They came across an art show put on by the local townspeople. The paintings in the show were the usual landscapes and still lifes. They were old-fashioned and unpretentious; however, they were pleasant, and some were beautiful. This dream might be captioned, "This is ordinary but I like it."

This patient, too, quickly understood his dream's meaning. He had always thought he would marry a woman like his mother, a former ballerina, who was flamboyant and charismatic. Now he was falling in love with a woman who was low-key, pleasant, and unpretentious. Just as in the dream he enjoyed the pleasant, unpretentious paintings, so in his everyday life he was enjoying his unpretentious, pleasant girlfriend. The patient relied on metaphor to give himself this message, because out of loyalty to his mother he was uncomfortable about giving it to himself directly.

The next dream, which occurred in the therapy of a man in his early 20s, told its story with the solemn authority of certain passages of the Old Testament.

> The patient dreamed that he was captured by a band of vigilantes, who punished him by cutting out his tongue. The dream could be captioned, "This is what you deserve."

In his associations, the patient remembered that in the previous session he had withheld a thought of which he was ashamed. It was that during masturbation he sometimes fantasized that he was a naughty child being spanked by a prim school teacher. The patient felt guilty about not revealing this fantasy. He equated not revealing it to lying, and he thought, "If I don't associate completely freely I will receive no help." In this dream, which alluded to castration, the dreamer was punished for lying by having his tongue cut out. By the severity of the punishment depicted in the dream, the patient revealed the extent to which he had complied with his moralizing father, a stern fundamentalist minister. In his dream the patient expressed guilt for not free-associating, and prodded himself by the threat of punishment to free-associate.

In the next example, the dreamer relied on the light-hearted mood of a sitcom to convey the dream's message. In this dream the patient referred to his relations with his wife, not directly, but by metaphor. The dreamer suffered unconsciously from an omnipotent sense of responsibility for women that stemmed from his belief in his mother's vulnerability. He was afraid to fight with his wife, even when she was clearly provocative. However, the night before the dream, the patient and his wife had quarreled, and the patient was relieved that both had emerged unscathed. In producing the dream, the dreamer emphasized the lesson he had learned from observing that his fighting with his wife did not endanger either of them.

> In the dream the patient and a companion, both armed with guns, bluffed their way past several guards into a forbidden building. The patient became frightened, and his gun, which was pointed at the plaster ceiling, went off. The patient then realized that his gun was only a BB gun. Nonetheless, the BBs shook a lot of plaster from the ceiling, which landed on the patient and his friend. Both burst out laughing, and the patient said, "Poor timing." The caption of the dream might be "The situation seemed ominous but was not."

In this dream the patient told himself that fighting with his wife was no more dangerous than shooting a BB gun at a plaster ceiling.

In another example, a patient, after a series of helpful therapy sessions, produced a dream in which he expressed a sense of exaltation that he was seeing his problems more clearly and putting them into perspective, and that he was ready to push forward with new accomplishments.

> In the dream, the patient was approaching San Francisco by ship. To either side of him was a vast armada of ships that reminded him of the Normandy invasion. The city was beautiful. The sky was various shades of gray with touches of orange and red. The stars and planets formed a ring of lights that seemed to make a halo over the city. As the patient approached the city, he explained to his son how the planets and stars were formed and why they were arranged in the form of a halo.

In the dream the patient used grandeur, beauty, and perspective to convey his sense of mastery, inspiration, and assurance.

THE ADAPTIVE FUNCTION OF REMEMBERING DREAMS

What determines whether a person remembers or forgets his dreams? Freud answered this question by reference to repression. He assumed that a person forgets his dreams in order to re-repress the mental contents expressed in them (1901, vol 5, p. 672), and he remembers his dreams when such repression fails to take place. I argue here that a person may remember his dreams, not simply when he fails to repress them, but when remembering them serves an adaptive function.

It seems that some dreams may perform their adaptive functions whether they are interpreted or even remembered (see Greenberg et al., 1992). However, there are circumstances when remembering a dream is essential to the dreamer's purpose. This applies to an engineer who, as described below, solved an important engineering problem in a series of dreams. I learned about the engineer's dreams from a letter he sent me after reading an article I wrote in a popular journal (Weiss, 1990), in which I stated that a person may solve problems unconsciously. I quote from the engineer's letter here, with minor changes in the interest of brevity and of disguising the dreamer's identity.

> I was born with a natural preference for the use of my left hand and was exclusively left-handed until I started school. At school the teachers forced me to use my right hand by slapping my left hand with a ruler when I used it for writing, drawing, and so forth. The teachers also convinced my parents to cooperate with them in making me right-handed.
>
> I am an engineer, 43 years of age, and am known as the father of a certain engineering process which is now widely used.
>
> In developing this process I relied on my dreams. When I perceived a problem in a device I was designing, I would think about it before I went to sleep, but would never find a solution. Then I would dream about the device. In the dream I would see the device go through part of its cycle correctly, but then stop at a certain point. I would wake up and realize that the design I visualized in the dream was not proper. I would think about it for about half an hour and then go back to sleep. Then, I would think about it again in the following night before sleeping. I would do this for weeks or months. Again I would dream of the device. I would depict its motions in fine detail. If the device was not working correctly, I would wake up and continue to think about the problem.
>
> I continued this process until, in my dreams, the device func-

tioned perfectly through its entire cycle. Then I would wake up and make a drawing of the device or build a model of it. The system I built in this way is now being used extensively.

All the concepts necessary to developing my process were first depicted for me in my dreams. Also, I rarely if ever woke up from dreams except when dreaming about my device.

Since the dreamer was not a patient, the dream process he described could not be examined in detail. The fact that the dreamer began his letter by reporting that he was forced in childhood to become right-handed provides a clue as to the meaning of his using dreams to solve an engineering problem. He may have inferred that he was not supposed to solve problems in a natural way. Since he was not permitted to use his left hand for writing or drawing, he did not permit himself to use his waking thoughts to solve his engineering problems. In any case, the engineer's dream makes clear that a person may unconsciously decide both to work on and to solve a particular technical problem in a dream, and also to wake up during the dream so as to remember the solution.

There are other circumstances when remembering dreams is essential to the dreamer's purpose. Remembering dreams is essential to the dreamer whose purpose in dreaming is to lift his repressions and bring forth traumatic memories. The former prisoners of war studied by Balson (1975), after their release from prison camp, all produced a series of vivid dreams in which they remembered the traumatic experiences of their capture and their mistreatments in the camp.

Patients in therapy who are working to remember traumatic experiences from childhood may behave like Balson's prisoners of war. Such patients during the beginning part of their therapies may scarcely remember their dreams. Then they may produce a series of dreams, which they remember vividly, and in which they retrieve the traumatic experiences. After they have become completely conscious of the experiences, they may, as at the beginning of treatment, remember only an occasional dream.

Such was the case in the therapy of a young woman who during the first 2 years of treatment scarcely remembered her dreams. Then, in the third year of her therapy, for a period of about 6 months, she produced a series of dreams that she remembered vividly. They were of her father, whom she consciously had always idealized. By means of these dreams, the patient gradually remembered a shocking experience involving her father when she was 8; it was of seeing him having sexual intercourse with the babysitter. After she brought her memories of this experience to consciousness, she continued therapy for another several years. However, during this last period of therapy as at the beginning, she remembered only an occasional dream.

Another kind of dream that the dreamer remembers for an adaptive purpose is the consoling dream that a person produces in dire circumstances. The power of these dreams to help the dreamer derives from their having the quality of real experience. For example, the captured soldiers, who dreamed that they were powerful and gratified reacted to the dreams as though they were in fact powerful and gratified. After such dreams they felt less helpless and more hopeful. Before producing these blissful dreams, the soldiers had tried to cheer themselves up in waking life by telling themselves that someday they would be free to gratify themselves, but they derived little comfort from these waking, wishful thoughts compared to the comfort they derived from the dreams.

In another example reported in Weiss et al. (1986, Chapter 7), a dream gave great comfort to a desperate patient. This patient was unloading his gun when it accidentally went off, killing his wife instantly. The patient, who loved his wife, became suicidal. In treating this patient, the therapist emphasized that the shooting was truly an accident; the patient realized that this was so, but nonetheless could not forgive himself. Then, about 8 months after beginning therapy, the patient dreamed that when he accidentally shot his wife she staggered over to him, fell on his lap, and told him that she forgave him. The dream, like the blissful dreams of the prisoners, was vivid, and it offered the patient great consolation. He remembered it for weeks afterward. When feeling depressed, he cheered himself up by going over it again. By producing the dream, the patient gave himself much greater consolation than he could give himself by waking thoughts. He reacted to the dream as though it had been a real experience—that is, as though his wife had in fact forgiven him.

WHAT THE THERAPIST MAY LEARN FROM THE PATIENT'S DREAMS

What Would the Patient Like to Face Consciously?

A person's dreams are never trivial (Freud, 1900). They are always about a pressing issue that he has not resolved by waking thought, sometimes because it is overwhelming. He then may attempt to deal with it both by conscious waking thought and in his dreams. This was the situation of the soldiers who feared capture, and of the soldiers mistreated in prison camp; it was also the situation of the man who accidentally killed his wife.

A person may also be unable to resolve a problem in his waking life because he is not ready to face it consciously. He may then take it up in his dreams. This is typically the case of the patient in psychotherapy: His dreams often reveal what he would like to discuss in his therapy, but is not quite ready to face. Indeed, his dreams may be constructed to alert the therapist to his preoccupations. Thus the therapist may learn from the patient's dreams what he would like to take up in his treatment.

Consider, for example, the patient whose dreams about blue ice females from outer space reduced to absurdity his fear of contamination by human females. The therapist assumed that the patient produced this dream because he had not yet overcome an identification with his mother's squeamishness, and so wanted help from the therapist in his efforts to overcome it. The therapist's assumption was borne out by the fact that the patient used the therapist's help to overcome this identification.

As another example, consider the patient who dreamed of liking unpretentious paintings in order to tell himself that he liked his unpretentious girlfriend. This dream alerted the therapist to the patient's wish to work in treatment to overcome his guilt about separating from his flamboyant mother.

The patient who dreamed that his tongue was cut out as a punishment for lying made the therapist aware of the great pressure the patient was experiencing from the therapist. The patient was perceiving the therapist as he had perceived his stern moralizing father. The therapist reacted by becoming more casual with the patient in an attempt to reduce the pressure the patient felt. The patient reacted well to this. He became less frightened of the therapist, could talk more freely to him, and brought out his fear of punishment by him.

The patient who produced a light-hearted dream of relief after discovering that fighting with his wife was not dangerous was using the dream to alert the therapist to his wanting to work in therapy on his fear of fighting with his wife.

A new example illustrates how the patient, a social worker, used a dream to tell himself that his fear of rejection was unfounded, and so alerted the therapist to his wanting to work in therapy on overcoming this fear.

> In the dream, the patient was driving his car when suddenly it was hit by a rock thrown by a young man driving in an adjoining lane. The patient decided to confront the young man and followed him to his house. There the young man jumped out of his car and quickly entered the house through the front door. The patient followed, rang the doorbell, and was greeted by the young man's mother. The patient introduced himself as a social worker and told the mother about the incident. He expected her to be angry and defend her son; however, she surprised the patient by being pleased and welcoming him into the house. She stated that she had been worried about her son's behavior and would like to discuss it with the patient. The dream might be captioned, "My fears were unfounded."

The patient quickly understood the meaning of the dream. He had been considering calling up a new girlfriend, but feared she would be annoyed. The dream, which relied on metaphor to carry its message, assured the patient that though he expected rejection, he might not receive it. The dream refocused the patient's and the therapist's attention on a familiar theme: the patient's fear of rejection from women, which stemmed from his relationship with his mother. During the rest of the hour, the patient remembered more about how his mother would sometimes react with annoyance when he tried to get her attention. The patient also realized that he had no reason to expect rejection from the girlfriend, and he called her soon afterward.

The next example is of a dream in which the patient reprimanded himself for being mean to his girlfriend. By this dream the patient alerted the therapist to his goal of becoming more reasonable with his girlfriend. The night before the dream, the girlfriend had complained mildly that the patient was becoming so busy that he was neglecting her. The patient took offense and his girlfriend apologized; however, the patient continued to pout even after the apology.

> In the dream, a friend informed the patient that his mother had died. He was chagrined that he had not been in touch with his mother and so had not known about her death.

The patient did in the dream what he failed to do in waking life: He accepted his girlfriend's accusation that he was too self-absorbed and self-righteous. He reprimanded himself for this. He told himself that such behavior was reprehensible, since it could lead to serious neglect of others as depicted in the dream. The therapist, alerted to the patient's goal of becoming more tolerant of his girlfriend, helped him to work toward this goal. This dream had the structure of a reduction-to-absurdity dream, in that it made its point by tracing the consequences of a particular attitude—namely, self-centeredness. However, it demonstrated, not that this attitude was absurd, but that it might be dangerous or destructive.

In the next example, a patient emphasized an idea that he found helpful and that he had recently applied in his work. It was that he was not responsible for the ways people behaved toward him. He thereby alerted the therapist that he wanted to work more in therapy on overcoming his pathogenic belief in his omnipotent responsibility for others. The patient, a clinical psychologist, had been treating a very disagreeable, almost impossible client, who had been blaming him in various ways for making her unhappy. Nothing the therapist did or said would satisfy her. The patient's supervisor helped the patient to get over feeling responsible for the client's unhappiness. The supervisor pointed out that the client was programmed to complain and would continue to complain no matter what the patient did. In his dream the next night, which was unusually well constructed, the patient generalized the idea that people are programmed, and he applied this idea to members of his family.

> In the dream, the patient was on a TV talk show in which the host was a right-wing conservative who liked to make fun of liberals. The patient, who was sitting next to a staff member of the show, had been hired to jeer at the guests. The first guests were two Harvard professors who were advocates of prison reform. Before either could speak, the host said, "I'd like to respond to you men," and launched into a tirade against prison reform. Next, a man in the front row dressed in prison stripes stood up, beat his chest, and said, "I'm an animal. I kill. I'm a beast." He was on the show to demonstrate that good treatment in prison is not helpful, for he had been receiving such treatment for years to no avail. After that, a sad social worker stood up and said apologetically, "I must admit that I am for prison reform."

The patient, after associating for about 10 minutes to the dream, explained that it was about the members of his family. It made clear to the patient how each had been programmed to behave in a particular way. The talk show host represented the patient's father, who talked a lot but did not listen to others. The man in prison stripes represented his brother, who was always crude and provocative. The sad social worker represented his mother, who was always sad and apologetic. By this dream the patient underlined the insight that since people's behaviors are programmed, he should not take so much responsibility for the way people behaved toward him. The patient was struggling to assure himself that he was not responsible for his father's rejecting him, his mother's complaining about him, or his brother's provocativeness.

In the next example, the patient produced a dream the

night before an analytic hour. It was intended to prepare her for the hour by showing her that her fear of offending the therapist was not warranted. Thus the dream threw light on the patient's relationship to the therapist.

> The patient dreamed that her baby son cried. She went to see why he was upset, found him covered with feces, and cleaned him. She added that she didn't mind cleaning him but that her husband did.

In the analytic hour that followed, the patient spent much of her time reporting sexual fantasies. She apologized for reveling in these fantasies, which she feared the therapist would find disgusting. In the dream the patient had attempted to reassure herself in advance that the therapist would not be offended. She told herself, "If I can tolerate cleaning my son's feces, the therapist can tolerate listening to my sexual fantasies." Her dream alerted the therapist to the patient's wish to focus more on her fear of offending others, including the therapist.

In still another example, a patient used a dream to bolster his resolve not to comply blindly with his girlfriend. He thereby alerted the therapist to his wish to work in therapy on the issue of blind compliance.

> The patient dreamed that a friend persuaded him to join him in robbing a bank. The two got away with it. However, they tried again, and the second time they were caught; the patient had to go to jail.

This dream, like reduction-to-absurdity dreams, made its point by tracing the consequences of a particular attitude—namely, blind obedience. It demonstrated that although such obedience is not necessarily absurd, it is dangerous. The dream might be captioned, "Don't comply as in the dream."

After the patient has resolved a previously unresolved issue by waking thought, he may stop dreaming about it. For example, a patient who in his waking thoughts trusted the analyst unconsciously feared that the analyst would betray him. Often, before his analytic sessions, he dreamed that he was being tricked and betrayed by an older man. By these dreams he warned himself of a danger of which he was not completely conscious. The patient stopped having such dreams after he realized consciously that he felt endangered by the analyst, and also that he had a right to protect himself from this danger.

In the final example of this section, a patient who had recently agreed with her therapist on a termination date dreamed that she had lost her cat. Her associations revealed that she had been worried that the therapist would feel sad about losing her, and in the dream she was putting herself in the therapist's place. Thus the dream threw light on an important part of the transference—namely, the patient's worry about the therapist's reaction to her termination.

Is the Therapist on the Right Track?

The therapist may check on the correctness of his approach to the patient by observing how the patient reacts to it, not only in his waking life, but also in his dreams. The patient by his dreams may affirm the correctness of an interpretation by agreeing with it, or by demonstrating more self-knowledge, or by expressing his feelings and ideas more freely.

This point may be illustrated by a dream in the therapy of Janice D., a patient presented in Chapter 4, who had been abused by her parents in childhood. She came to therapy for the purpose of obtaining support for not going back to her abusive husband. The patient disliked her previous therapist, a male psychiatrist, who told her that she was recreating in her marriage the situation of her childhood. She experienced this interpretation as blaming her for the abuse she had received from her husband, and thus as confirming her pathogenic belief that she deserved the abuse. After the patient's second therapist, a female social worker, told the patient that she had not provoked her husband's abuse and did not deserve it, the patient had a happy dream.

> She dreamed that she had come to a hospital to have a scalp wound treated. A clumsy physician had botched an

earlier attempt to treat it. However, a pleasant nurse practitioner would now help the patient heal it.

By this dream the patient revealed, through the use of metaphor, that she had disliked the first therapist, but liked her new therapist and was helped by her interpretations. The patient thereby confirmed that the new therapist was on the right track. This dream made clear to the therapist that the patient was still trying to convince herself that she had been mistreated by her first therapist. If the patient had already been convinced of this, she would not have been motivated to produce a dream in which she told herself how much she preferred the new therapist.

In another example, a patient revealed in her dream that the therapist had been passing her tests. The dream occurred in the analysis of a patient who had become aware in therapy that she had been sexually abused by her father, and that her father had denied the abuse. For several sessions before producing the dream, the patient had been testing the therapist by describing her misery and implying the possibility of suicide. The therapist had responded by conveying that she was quite concerned about the patient, but would not be paralyzed or rendered incompetent by worry about her.

> In the dream, the patient was an adolescent exploring a dense forest with a group of other adolescents. They discovered a completely abandoned village. The houses were all made of white plaster. The sun was shining. It was very hot, but there were no shadows. They entered a large house and found a box of sparkling jewelry. The others were intrigued. They believed the jewelry was valuable. However, the patient knew it was worthless.

The dream's surrealistic atmosphere suggested dark secrets. However, as the patient's associations made clear, its primary message was the patient's complaint, conveyed by metaphor and symbol, that her father's sexually abusing her had prevented her from enjoying her adolescence. It had kept her from sharing in her friends' pleasure and excitement in the discovery of sex, and thereby had caused her to be alienated.

Previously, the patient had scarcely allowed herself to complain even in her dreams that her father had damaged her. She suffered from the pathogenic belief that she was omnipotently responsible for him, and she feared that if she complained about his abuse of her, she would kill him. In therapy the patient worked to change the belief in her responsibility for her father by testing it through turning passive into active. She behaved as though the therapist were responsible for her happiness, and even for keeping her alive. By implication she blamed the therapist for her depression and thoughts of suicide. The therapist passed the patient's test by being concerned about her without accepting the responsibility the patient was thrusting on her. The therapist thereby provided the patient with a model of someone who did not feel omnipotent. The patient, by identifying with the therapist, took a step toward changing her pathogenic belief in her own omnipotence. She gained confidence that her complaining about her father would not kill him, and so she permitted herself to complain about him indirectly in her dream.

THE VALUE OF DREAM INTERPRETATION

The importance of dream interpretation varies from patient to patient. Some patients never report dreams, or report them very rarely. In such patients, the occasional dream may or may not be especially informative.

An instance in which the patient produced only one dream in a long psychotherapy has been discussed in Chapter 5. It occurred in the therapy of Margaret M., and helped the therapist to understand how he could help Margaret. As described earlier, the patient was a 70-year-old woman who in childhood had given a great deal to her depressed mother while receiving little in return, and who had continued throughout life to give without receiving. For a number of years Margaret had suffered from paranoid delusions. Since she assumed the therapist received payment from the state for her psychotherapy, she believed that she was cheating the state and that she would be severely punished for this, perhaps by execution.

The therapist, who saw the patient for only 20 minutes per week, had not been billing the state for the therapy, for it would have cost him more to bill the state than he would have received in payment. The therapist had been reluctant to tell the patient that he was not being paid for treating her; he feared she would believe she was cheating him. However, on one occasion when the patient expressed worry about cheating the state, the therapist reconsidered and told the patient that from then on he would not charge her for her treatment.

> On her next visit, Margaret reported a dream in which she was in a small wooden hut by herself, situated on a plain. A storm raged outside, and the ground around her was covered with snow. The patient heard a thud outside and assumed that it was caused by her mother's falling down. The patient rushed to the door, opened it, and was relieved to see that no one was there. She would not be burdened by her responsibility for her mother.

The dream made clear that the therapist's telling the patient he would not charge her did not increase her guilt; rather, it reduced it. Apparently the patient took the therapist's offer as meaning that she deserved his help. She could assume the role of the recipient, rather than her usual role of the giver. The dream made the therapist realize that by giving to her he was helping her to disconfirm the belief that she was undeserving. He began to give her small inexpensive presents. She enjoyed receiving them and was helped to feel a little more self-esteem.

Occasionally a patient produces such lucid dreams and is so good at dream interpretation that the therapist may base his hypotheses about the patient mainly on his understanding of the patient's dreams. Indeed, a dream may occasionally reveal a patient's plans and goals so clearly that it constitutes a royal road to the patient's unconscious. However, as already noted, most dreams are not transparent. Dream interpretation is often difficult, and many dreams remain obscure.

Fortunately, a therapist need not rely on dream interpretation to infer the patient's pathogenic beliefs, plans, and goals. Indeed, in attempting to infer them, the therapist, as described in Chapter 4, should take account of everything he knows about the patient, including the patient's reactions to the therapist. The therapist, in treating a patient who does not dream, may stay on track by keeping in mind that the patient seldom makes changes in his basic plans. He works for long periods of time, perhaps years, to disprove one or two major pathogenic beliefs and to pursue one or two major goals.

SUMMARY

In this chapter I have tried to show that a patient's dreams deal with his current concerns; that they carry a simple message to the dreamer; and that in making their messages clear they rely on techniques familiar from conscious waking life, as well as from art and poetry. The therapist and the patient may learn from the patient's dreams what problems the patient is working on in therapy, how he is perceiving the therapist, and how he wants the therapist to help him.

RESEARCH AND A COMPARISON OF THEORIES

CHAPTER 8

THE EMPIRICAL BASIS
OF THE THEORY

This chapter presents research studies that offer strong support for the views proposed in this book. The studies were done by the Mount Zion Psychotherapy Research Group, which I co-direct with Harold Sampson. Our method was to test the explanatory power of fundamental hypotheses about unconscious mental functioning, psychopathology, and psychotherapy. This method has enabled us to test major hypotheses that, as I discuss below, cannot be tested clinically. Thus it has enabled us to choose between competing hypotheses.

Our research[1] demonstrates that the theory of therapy and technique presented here is powerful. It enables us to make relatively accurate predictions about the course of events in small segments of therapy, and about the course and outcome of an entire treatment.

RESEARCH METHODS

In doing research, the Mount Zion group uses reliable data—namely, the transcripts of entire therapies that have been re-

[1]Our research has been supported by National Institute of Mental Health Grant Nos. MH-13915, MH-34052, and MH-35230. Also, we have received administrative help and financial support from the Mount Zion Hospital and Medical Center. In addition, we have received grants from the Fund for Psychoanalytic Research, the Broitman Foundation, and the Miriam F. Meehan Charitable Trusts.

corded on audiotape for research purposes. The group uses rating scales to measure a wide variety of phenomena about patients and therapists. Such scales permit investigators to make subtle discriminations. For example, independent raters using such scales can agree on slight changes in a patient's level of anxiety or defensiveness, or on the degree to which the therapist is attuned to a particular patient at a particular time.

We use blind judgments in order to prevent raters from being biased by expectations; that is, the information offered to each rater contains no extraneous information that could influence his ratings. Also, we use statistics to determine the reliability of our measures, to quantify the relationships between variables, and to indicate the significance of findings.

THE PROPOSITIONS AND THE RESEARCH THAT SUPPORTS THEM

In this chapter, I present a series of propositions that our research supports. Also, I indicate briefly how the research supporting each proposition was carried out, and how the findings pertain to the theory of technique.

Proposition I

The patient in therapy exerts control over his repressions. He may and often does lift his repressions and bring previously warded-off mental contents to consciousness without these contents having been interpreted. He brings them forth when he unconsciously decides that he can safely experience them. Thus, their emergence may be undramatic and nonconflictual.

This first proposition is of great importance for both theory and practice. Yet observations supporting it are seldom reported by clinicians. A notable exception is contained in the work of Ernst Kris (1956b), who stated that a patient, before becoming conscious of a mental content, may prepare himself unconsciously to experience it, and then bring it forth in an undramatic way that is unlikely to attract the attention of the therapist. That is, he may bring it forth without conflict and without acknowledging that it was previously repressed.

Why have clinicians failed to observe this? For one thing, its regular occurrence runs counter to the theory that Freud presented in the *Papers on Technique* (1911–1915). As noted in Chapter 9, this theory assumes that the patient neither controls his repressions nor is motivated to lift them. In general, he becomes conscious of a repressed mental content only if it is interpreted. Thus a clinician who subscribes to Freud's early theory and who observes a patient talking easily about a particular mental content assumes that the content was not previously repressed.

Even if his observations are not guided by theory, the clinician is unlikely to observe the nonconflictual emergence of previously repressed mental contents. To do so he would have to make careful formulations about what mental contents were repressed at the beginning of treatment, and then to note when and how these contents became conscious. For the clinician this would be a difficult and unnecessary task. Yet it is a task readily carried out by the investigator who uses careful research methods and whose verbatim transcripts he and others may study at leisure, untroubled by the drama of the unfolding treatment.

The starting point for our investigation of the patient's control of his repressions was our clinical impression, derived from the reading of process notes, that a patient frequently does bring forth previously repressed mental contents that have not been interpreted. Suzanne Gassner formally tested this proposition in the transcripts of the first 100 sessions in the analysis of Mrs. C. (Gassner, Sampson, Weiss, & Brumer, 1982). Gassner knew from previous studies that Mrs. C. made considerable progress during these 100 sessions, despite the analyst's relatively few interpretations. Gassner therefore assumed that if in fact previously warded-off contents do come forth without interpretation, she should find such contents in these sessions.

Gassner used an ingenious method. Rather than attempting to locate repressed contents in the first 10 therapy sessions and then attempting to determine which of these contents become conscious in the later sessions, she did the reverse. She first had judges study the transcripts of the first 100 sessions, to locate all contents contained in these sessions but not contained in sessions 1–40. She then had a number of independent judges study these contents, along with the process notes of the first 10 sessions, to determine whether any of the contents had been repressed at the beginning of treatment. The judges found that a substantial number of the contents had been repressed at the beginning of treatment, and they agreed about which contents these were.

Gassner's next task was to eliminate from the study any contents that had been interpreted prior to their emergence. She did this by having a list of all the previously repressed mental contents compared with a list of all the therapist's interpretations. It turned out that all but one of the previously repressed contents came forth without having been interpreted. This finding is important in its own right. It shows that the patient may bring forth previously repressed mental contents on his own, without benefit of interpretation.

Now Gassner's task was to determine why and how the uninterpreted contents came forth. She considered the following three explanations, the first two of which are based on the "automatic-functioning hypothesis" (AFH) and the third (our proposition) on the "higher-mental-functioning hypothesis" (HMFH) (see Chapters 1 and 9):

1. Previously repressed contents may come forth because they are intensified, so that they push through the patient's repressions to consciousness.
2. The contents may come forth because they are disguised, so that their importance is not recognized and they escape detection by the repressing forces.
3. The contents may come forth because the patient unconsciously decides that he can safely experience them, and so lifts the repressions opposing them and brings them forth.

The three hypotheses make different and testable predictions about (1) how anxious the patient will feel as the contents emerge and (2) how much he will experience them. To experience mental contents means to focus on them, to reflect on them, and to use them constructively, as opposed to being defensively uninvolved with them.

If a content comes forth by pushing through the patient's repressions, the patient will come into conflict with it while it is emerging, and so will become anxious. However, the degree to which he will experience the content cannot be predicted. (Prediction: high anxiety, no prediction about experiencing.)

If a content emerges because it is disguised so that its import is not recognized, the patient will not react to its emergence, so that he will not become anxious about it. Also, since it is isolated, he will not fully experience it. (Prediction: low anxiety, low experiencing.)

If a content emerges because the patient unconsciously decides that he can safely experience it and so lifts his defenses against it, he will have overcome his anxiety about it before bringing it forth. Therefore, he will not feel anxious about it and will be able fully to experience it. (Prediction: low anxiety, high experiencing.)

Which prediction best fits the data? Gassner's next step was to use measurements to determine this. She had two sets of judges (raters) use rating scales to measure how anxious the patient felt while the contents were emerging. One set of judges used the Mahl scale (Mahl, 1956); the other used the Gottschalk–Gleser scale (Gottschalk, 1974). She had a third set of judges use the Experiencing scale (Klein, Mathieu, Gendlin, & Kiesler, 1970) to measure how fully the patient experienced what she was saying while the contents were coming forth.

Gassner's findings supported our proposition (the third hypothesis above). While the contents were emerging the patient was not especially anxious, and according to the Mahl scale, she was less anxious than in random segments—a statistically significant finding. Also, Mrs. C. did experience things fully while the contents were emerging. Indeed, she experienced the emerging contents more fully than she experienced random segments, and this finding was also statistically significant.

The implications of these findings (which are consistent with the findings of other studies reported below) are far-reaching and have been discussed throughout this book. As already noted, the findings indicate that interpretation is not the sine qua non of therapy. A person may make progress and develop insights without interpretation (as our other studies also show). Our findings support the thesis that the analyst should create conditions that make it safe for the patient to work at mastering his problems. The patient may then make progress on his own. He may, among other things, bring forth and constructively experience previously repressed mental contents, unaided by interpretation.

Proposition II
   Throughout therapy the patient tests his pathogenic beliefs in relation to the therapist, in an effort to disconfirm the beliefs.

The starting point for our investigation of this proposition was our clinical impression, gained from the study of the process notes of Mrs. C.'s analysis, that throughout her therapy she tested her pathogenic beliefs in relation to the analyst. She made demands on the analyst to test her omnipotent belief that she could force him to do whatever she wanted. She experienced the analyst as passing her tests when he did not yield to her demands—that is, when he maintained analytic neutrality. When he passed her tests by not yielding, Mrs. C. made progress by becoming bolder and more insightful.

This observation intrigued us because it indicated that in the analysis of Mrs. C., the attitude of analytic neutrality recommended by the 1911–1915 theory was helpful. In many cases it is not; often it is harmful. Suppose, for example, that a patient tests the therapist by being self-destructive, in the hope of assuring himself that the therapist will attempt to protect him from his self-destructiveness. In this circumstance analytic neutrality would be a highly inadequate response, because the patient would infer from it that the therapist was unconcerned about him.

According to our clinical impression, by not yielding to her demands the analyst helped Mrs. C. in her efforts to disprove the belief, inferred in relation to her volatile and vulnerable parents, that by making demands on an authority she would upset him. Mrs. C. tested this belief by making demands, and was helped to disprove it by the analyst's not yielding to her demands.

The observation that Mrs. C., unlike many patients, benefited from analytic neutrality suggested a research project: We could compare our hypothesis about why Mrs. C made demands on the analyst to the 1911–1915 hypothesis derived from the 1911–1915 theory. According to our hypothesis (the HMFH), Mrs. C. made demands on the analyst to test her pathogenic beliefs. She was helped by the analyst's neutrality, because by being neutral the analyst passed her tests and so helped her in her efforts to disprove the beliefs. As she succeeded in disproving these beliefs, she unconsciously decided that she could bring forth previously repressed contents.

According to the 1911–1915 hypothesis (the AFH), Mrs. C. made unconscious demands on the analyst to gratify unconscious impulses. The analyst's neutrality was helpful because it frustrated these impulses, thereby intensifying them and bringing them closer to the surface.

Both hypotheses agree that the therapist should not have yielded to Mrs. C.'s demands, and both predict that she would have benefited from his not yielding. However, the two hypotheses make different predictions about how the patient would have reacted immediately following the analyst's not yielding to her demands. According to our hypothesis, Mrs. C. should have been relieved when the analyst remained unyielding. She should have become less anxious, more relaxed, and bolder. According to the 1911–1915 hypothesis, Mrs. C. should have reacted in the opposite way: Since her unconscious impulses were frustrated, she should have become more tense and anxious.

Silberschatz (1986) tested the two hypotheses against each other by determining how Mrs. C. did in fact react when she experienced the analyst as not yielding to her unconscious demands. Silberschatz took special pains to ensure that his research design would be fair to both hypotheses. He devised his research plan with the help of two senior consultants, one of whom subscribed to the 1911–1915 theory (the AFH), and the other to our theory (the HMFH). The procedure he designed was satisfactory to both consultants.

Silberschatz's first step was to locate in the transcripts of the first 100 sessions of Mrs. C.'s analysis a large number of interactions in which Mrs. C. made a powerful unconscious demand on the analyst. He then honed this list so that it would include only those demands that fit the criteria of both hypotheses—that is, demands that could be construed either as attempts to gratify an important unconscious impulse, or as attempts to test an important pathogenic belief. Silberschatz did this by asking judges who subscribed to the AFH to identify instances in which Mrs. C. was attempting to gratify an important unconscious impulse, and by asking judges who subscribed to the HMFH to identify instances in which Mrs. C. was unconsciously giving an important test. He then selected for further study those interactions that satisfied both groups of judges—that is, the overlap group.

Silberschatz studied the patient–therapist interactions in this overlap group by having yet another set of judges rate the therapist's responses to the demands the patient unconsciously made on him. He asked judges who subscribed to the AFH to rate each analytic response for how well the response frustrated the patient's unconscious impulses. He asked judges accustomed to thinking in terms of the HMFH to decide how well the responses passed Mrs. C.'s unconscious tests. This procedure enabled Silberschatz to distinguish between interventions that frustrated Mrs. C.'s impulses or passed her tests, and interventions that did not frustrate her impulses or pass her tests. The procedure also enabled Silberschatz to correlate the findings of the two sets of judges, and thus to demonstrate that the interventions seen by one set of judges as frustrating Mrs. C.'s unconscious impulses were the ones seen by the other set of judges as passing her unconscious tests.

Silberschatz's next task was to determine how Mrs. C. reacted to the analyst's nonyielding responses by determining how her behavior changed from just before such a response to just after it. He asked judges to rate segments of Mrs. C.'s speech from just before and from just after each of the analyst's responses. The speech segments were rated on scales designed to assess Mrs. C.'s levels of boldness, anxiety, relaxation, and loving feelings. The judges were blind as to whether a segment came before or after an analytic response and as to which analytic session it came from. Silberschatz then calculated the shifts in the patient's behavior from before an analytic response to after it, as determined by a comparison between the pre-response segments and the corresponding postresponse segments. (He used a statistical method that yielded a residualized gain score.)

The findings revealed that when the analyst did not yield to Mrs. C.'s unconscious demands, and therefore either passed her tests or frustrated her impulses, Mrs. C. became less anxious, bolder, more relaxed, and more loving (we assume that she became more loving because she appreciated the analyst's favorable responses). These findings were statistically significant, and they demonstrate that Mrs. C. was not frustrated but relieved when the analyst remained neutral in the face of her demands.

The study reported in connection with Proposition I (the Gassner study) demonstrated that during the first 100 sessions of her analysis, Mrs. C. brought forth a number of previously warded-off mental contents without their having been interpreted. While she was becoming conscious of these contents, Mrs. C. was feeling less anxious and experiencing things more fully than usual. We inferred from this that she brought these contents forth because she had unconsciously overcome her anxiety about them, and so had decided that she could safely experience them. The Silberschatz study indicates how Mrs. C. may unconsciously have overcome her anxiety about the contents without their having been interpreted. She may have done this by testing her pathogenic beliefs, and by such testing may have made progress in disconfirming these beliefs.

In sum, the Silberschatz study supports the following proposition: If, as in the case of Mrs. C., the analyst's neutrality helps the patient bring forth new material, this is not because it frustrates the patient or weakens his defenses. Rather, it is because it reassures the patient and thus enables him to feel safe enough to tolerate material he was previously afraid to experience.

Proposition III:

   Throughout therapy the patient works with the therapist at the task of disconfirming his unconscious pathogenic beliefs. He works in accordance with an unconscious plan for disconfirming them, and does so in two different ways: (1) by testing the beliefs in relation to the therapist in the hope of disconfirming them, and (2) by using the therapist's interpretations to become aware of the beliefs and to realize that they are false and maladaptive. Thus the therapist may help the patient either by passing the patient's tests or by offering him interpretations that he can use in his struggle to disconfirm the beliefs.

   The demonstration of this proposition required numerous interrelated studies. These studies, unlike the two studies reported so far, were designed not to compare the explanatory power of the AFH and HMFH, but to show that concepts derived from the HMFH bring a high degree of order, clarity, and predictability to the understanding of the therapeutic process. Since these studies assumed a reliable formulation of the patient's unconscious plan, our first step was to demonstrate that raters familiar with the transcripts of the first few sessions of a therapy (while blind to the others) could agree in their formulations of the patient's plan. To do this required us to find a way of comparing clinical formulations.

   Caston (1986) assumed that formulations written in narrative style would be difficult if not impossible to compare. He solved the problem of comparing formulations by an innovative method: He broke down the plan formulation into four components. These were (1) the patient's goals, (2) the obstacles (pathogenic beliefs) that prevented the patient from pursuing his goals, (3) the tests that the patient carried out in his efforts to disconfirm the beliefs, and (4) the insights that the patient found useful in his efforts to do this. Instead of having each rater write his own formulations of these components in narrative form, Caston presented each rater with a large inclusive list of Mrs. C.'s possible goals, pathogenic beliefs, tests, and insights, along with the transcripts of the first 10 sessions. Caston asked each judge first to read the transcripts, and then to rate each item for the degree to which it was pertinent to the patient's plan. Finally, he used statistical methods to determine the degree to which the independent raters agreed with one another. He demonstrated a high level of agreement. As of this writing, using Caston's method with certain revisions (Curtis & Silberschatz, 1986; Silberschatz & Curtis, 1986; Rosenberg, Silberschatz, Curtis, Sampson, & Weiss, 1986), we have studied 4 analyses and 10 brief psychotherapies and have found that the raters agreed reliably about the patient's plan in each case.

Once we demonstrated that we were able to develop reliable plan formulations from the transcripts of the first few sessions of a case, we had in hand a powerful tool for studying the subsequent sessions. We then used our plan formulations to study both the patients' testing of the therapist and the patients' use of the therapist's interpretations.

I illustrate our method by describing a series of studies carried out by Polly .Fretter (1984), Jessica Broitman (1985), and Lynn Davilla (1992) on the effects of interpretation in three brief psychotherapies. In these studies,[2] Fretter, Broitman, and Davilla tested the hypothesis that a patient would demonstrate immediate benefit from pro-plan interpretations, but not from anti-plan or irrelevant interpretations.

To test this hypothesis, Fretter first located in the transcripts of three brief therapies all the therapists' interpretations. Then she gave a team of independent judges the list of interpretations and the plan formulation for each patient, and she had each judge rate each interpretation for how planful (plan-compatible) it was. The judges rated the interpretations on a 5-point rating scale ranging from "strongly anti-plan" to "strongly pro-plan."

Fretter then had an independent set of judges rate each patient's level of experiencing in segments of the patient's speech occurring immediately before and immediately after each interpretation. The judges were blind both to the interpretations and to whether the speech segments occurred before the interpretations or after them. Fretter now correlated the shift in the patient's level of experiencing from before each

---

[2]The studies were carried out under the supervision of Curtis and Silberschatz.

interpretation to after it with the degree to which the interpretation was pro-plan. She demonstrated in each case that the more pro-plan the interpretation, the greater the shift in a progressive direction in the patient's level of experiencing. This finding was statistically significant. The correlation between the mean planfulness (plan compatibility) of the interpretations during each therapy hour and the mean shift in the patient's level of experiencing during that hour ranged for the three cases from .60 to .80 (Silberschatz, Fretter, & Curtis, 1986).

Broitman (1985) and Davilla (1992) studied the same patients, the same interpretations, and the same speech segments as Fretter had studied. Broitman demonstrated a statistically significant correlation between the planfulness of the therapist's interpretations and immediate shifts in the patient's level of insight as measured by a generic insight scale (the Morgan Patient Insight Scale). Davilla demonstrated that in two of the three cases the patient, after a pro-plan interpretation, moved toward his goals as defined in the patient's plan formulations (the third patient did not). This finding was statistically significant. Fretter's, Broitman's, and Davilla's findings all support our hypothesis.

In a number of studies of the patient's unconscious testing, we demonstrated a statistically significant correlation between (1) the degree to which the therapist's response to a test was pro-plan (i.e., the degree to which the therapist passed the patient's test), and (2) the shift in a progressive direction from before to after the therapist's response to the test. We studied a number of patients and used a variety of scales to measure this shift. In a study of one patient, we demonstrated that after a passed test the patient showed more pro-plan insight (as defined by the patient's plan formulation) than immediately before the test (Linsner, 1987). In another study of two patients (Silberschatz & Curtis, in press), we demonstrated that immediately after a passed test the patient showed a higher level of experiencing than just before the passed test. One of the patients also showed an immediate increase in boldness; the other did not. In a study of three cases, we demonstrated that in two of the three cases the patient reacted to a passed test by demonstrating an immediate decrease in tension, as measured by the Voice Stress Measure (Kelly, 1989). In a study of one patient, we demonstrated that immediately after a passed test the patient demonstrated a greater capacity to exert control over regressive behavior (Bugas, 1986).

The above-cited studies are of far-reaching significance for both the theoretician and the clinician. They provide strong support for our propositions about the patient's unconscious plan, his testing of the therapist, and his use of the therapist's interpretations. These propositions bring clarity to the therapeutic process. They offer the therapist a relatively simple but powerful guide to technique. They strongly support the recommendations that the therapist infer the patient's unconscious plan for disconfirming his pathogenic beliefs; that the therapist use his knowledge of the patient's unconscious plan to recognize the patient's tests; and that, if possible, he pass the tests. In addition, the therapist should offer the patient interpretations that may help him carry out his plan.

Moreover, our findings provide the clinician with a useful criterion for evaluating his approach. If the patient responds to the therapist's behavior, attitudes, or interpretations with relief, decreased anxiety, greater openness, and movement toward his goals, the therapist is probably on the right track. If, on the other hand, the patient responds by becoming anxious, more defensive, and bogged down, the therapist is probably off track.

Our finding that the patient responds immediately either to passed tests or to pro-plan interpretations by demonstrating a decrease in anxiety and an increase in both insight and experiencing is of considerable theoretical importance. It indicates that the patient is continually assessing the therapist to determine whether and to what extent he may rely on the therapist not to endanger him, and that the patient continually regulates his behavior in accordance with these assessments. He becomes more relaxed and open when he feels safe; and he becomes more tense and anxious when he feels in danger. This is highly compatible with Freud's formulation (1940a, p. 199), that the patient unconsciously tests reality and regulates his behavior in accordance with his assessment of his current reality.

Proposition IV

The higher the proportion of pro-plan interpretations the therapist offers the patient during therapy, the better the patient will do at outcome.

This proposition has been supported by two studies of brief time-limited (16-session) psychotherapy. The first was done by Fretter (1984) under the supervision of Curtis and Silberschatz (Silberschatz et al., 1986), using the same three therapies on which she studied the immediate effects of interpretation. She found in her small sample that the higher the percentage of pro-plan interpretations the therapist gave the patient, the better the patient did at outcome. The patient's outcome was determined 6 months after the termination of therapy by clinical interviews and by the use of extensive generic (non-case-specific) outcome measures. The patient who did the best at outcome was given interpretations that were 89% pro-plan, 2% anti-plan, and the rest ambiguous. The patient who did next best was given interpretations that were 80% pro-plan and 20% anti-plan. The patient who did the least well was given interpretations that were 50% pro-plan, 44% ambiguous, and 6% anti-plan. Using similar methods, Fretter demonstrated that transference interpretations are no more effective than non-transference interpretations. That is, patients who were given a high proportion of transference interpretations did no better at outcome than patients who were not.

The second study supporting our proposition about the relationship of interpretations to outcome was done by Norville (1989), who studied seven brief psychotherapy cases (16 sessions each; these included the three cases studied by Fretter). Norville isolated all of the interpretations offered each patient in five sessions. We selected these sessions as follows: We divided the last 15 sessions of each therapy into 5 groups of 3 sessions each; one such group consisted of sessions 2, 3, and 4, another of sessions 5, 6, and 7, and so forth. We then randomly selected a session in each group of 3.

In her list of interpretations, Norville included only as much of the patient's speech prior to the interpretation as was needed to make the context of the interpretation clear. For each case, she then had a number of independent judges who were familiar with the patient's plan use a scale to rate each interpretation for its degree of planfulness. The judges were in high agreement, as determined statistically. Norville then calculated the mean planfulness (plan compatibility) of the interpretations for each of the 5 hours studied, and, in addition, the mean for all 5 hours. She correlated this overall mean with the outcome as determined 6 months after termination. She found that in six of the seven cases, the mean of the ratings for plan compatibility was highly related to outcome.

The studies reported above provide additional support for the plan concept. They alert the therapist to the importance of inferring the patient's plan and of using his knowledge of the plan to make helpful (plan-compatible) interpretations. They suggest that the criterion most important for judging interpretations is plan compatibility.

Proposition V

The patient who knows in advance that he will be given only a limited number of sessions unconsciously plans his therapy in accordance with this knowledge. His purpose is to use the limited number of sessions as efficiently as possible.

The starting point for our investigation of this proposition was our clinical impression that the patient makes his pathogenic beliefs, goals, and plans clear to the therapist at the beginning of therapy, in order to provide the therapist with the knowledge he will need to pass the patient's tests. The patient then appears to lose insight, and makes false statements about himself in order to test the therapist. He hopes that the therapist will remember his plans, and will supply the missing insights and refute the false statements.

We decided to test this clinical impression by tracing the patient's level of insight throughout therapies that the patient knew in advance would be time-limited. The study was carried out on the transcripts of four patients who had agreed in advance to limit their therapies to 16 sessions (Edelstein, 1992; O'Connor, Edelstein, Berry, & Weiss, submitted for publication; Weiss, in press). In each case, we studied the transcripts of the intake interview (carried out by an independent evaluator), the patient's 16 sessions with his therapist, a posttherapy interview (carried out on completion of therapy by the independent evaluator), and a follow-up interview carried out 6 months after the completion of therapy (again by the independent evaluator).

Our method was straightforward. The investigators' first step was to have several judges, each of whom was provided with a formulation of the patient's plan, extract from the transcripts of each of the four therapies all the patient's statements in which he showed useful (pro-plan) insights. The investigators then presented a list of these insight statements in random order to four raters, who also were provided with a formulation of each patient's plan. In addition, the raters received a 5-point scale for rating each statement for the degree to which the insight it contained was pro-plan.

In compiling our findings, we calculated the degree of insight in each session by adding up the ratings of each insight statement for that session. In each case, the patient's level of insight followed a similar pattern, which was congruent with our clinical impression. Each patient demonstrated a moderate degree of pro-plan insight in the intake interview, and three patients, Rachel, Robert, and Irene, demonstrated even more pro-plan insight in the first therapy session. The fourth patient, Hilde, demonstrated considerable pro-plan insight in her third session.

Each patient then appeared to lose insight. Rachel had no pro-plan insights in session 11; Robert in sessions 5 and 12; Irene in sessions 6, 7, 8, 10 and 14, and Hilde in sessions 8, 12, 13, 14 and 15. The three patients who remained in therapy showed some pro-plan insight in their last session; the fourth, Robert, stopped in an unplanned way before the end of the therapy. Each patient showed considerable insight in the posttherapy session conducted by the independent evaluator. Two of the four showed high insight in their 6-month follow-up sessions with the independent evaluator; one showed moderate insight; and one showed poor insight. In each case, a graph of the patient's level of insight from the intake session through the 6-month follow-up session approximated a parabola: It was high at the beginning and at the end, but low in the middle. The approximation to a parabola is statistically significant (see Figure 8.1).[3]

Here is our explanation for these findings. During the intake interview with the independent evaluator, each patient revealed a moderate degree of insight because he came to therapy with a specific problem. He had thought about this problem and had developed some self-knowledge about it. Then, at the beginning of his work with the therapist, the patient demonstrated even more insight: At this starting point, he was highly motivated to give the therapist the information that the therapist would need to help him. The patient then tested his pathogenic beliefs with the therapist by appearing to lose insight and by making false statements about himself, in the hope that the therapist would supply the missing insights and refute the false statements. As the therapist passed the patient's tests, the patient became more secure with the therapist. His realization that the therapist disagreed with his pathogenic beliefs and was sympathetic to his goals encouraged the patient to test the therapist more vigorously—that is, by appearing to lose more insight. Toward the middle of the 16 sessions, the patient appeared to lose all pro-plan insight. However, as he came close to finishing the therapy, he became afraid of testing the therapist too vigorously. He did not want to finish therapy still testing the therapist by having little or no insight into his goals; therefore, he stopped testing vigorously and once again demonstrated a higher level of pro-plan insight.

These points may be illustrated by the example of Rachel. She strongly implied in the intake interview and in her first therapy session that she wanted to become more separate from her comatose, dying husband, and to get a job, but that she was impeded by a sense of guilt. Later she tried to determine wheth-

---

[3]In a fifth therapy that was studied after this book was written, the patient also lost insight during the course of her therapy. However, a parabolic curve did not significantly fit the raw scores due to greater variability in insight throughout the therapy. The plot of smoothed scores, however, indicated that the pattern was also parabolic, though less dramatically so. The quadratic regression closely approached significance ($p = .052$ for the quadratic term in the regression).

LEVEL OF INSIGHT

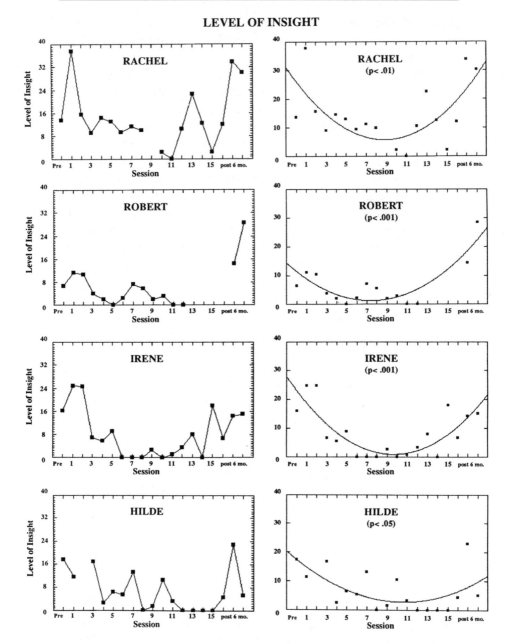

FIGURE 8.1. Graphs of four patients' levels of insight in brief time-limited (16-session) psychotherapy, from the intake session through the 6-month follow-up.

er the therapist approved of this goal by testing him: She appeared to lose her pro-plan insight, and she raised objections to finding a job by stating that she was untrained for work. The therapist passed her tests by supplying her missing pro-plan insights and by refuting her objections to working. Then, toward the end of therapy, the patient stopped testing her therapist, so she again displayed more insight.

Each patient revealed more insight in the posttherapy session and in the 6-month follow-up session than during the low points in his therapy. The reason for this may have been that in these interviews, the patient saw an independent evaluator, not a therapist; since the purpose of seeing the evaluator was not therapy, the patient did not test the evaluator and so demonstrated more insight.

The study reported above shows a close relationship between (1) the plan compatibility of the interpretations that the patient received; (2) the degree of insight he demonstrated in the follow-up interviews; and (3) the outcome of the therapy as assessed by the patient, the independent evaluator, and the therapist, and also as indicated by a group of non-case-specific outcome measures that were completed by the patient. The two patients who received the most pro-plan interpretations, Robert and Rachel, showed the most insight in their follow-up interviews and had the best outcomes. Irene, who received moderately good interpretations, showed a moderate degree of insight in her follow-up interviews and had a moderately good outcome. Hilde, who received poor interpretations, showed little insight in her follow-up interviews and had a poor outcome. Hilde's low insight during the middle and later parts of her therapy may have expressed not testing, but compliance with false (anti-plan) interpretations.

As discussed above, a patient who is given pro-plan interpretations during his 16-session psychotherapy may not demonstrate much more insight at the end of treatment than at the beginning. Nonetheless, he may, according to the present theory, be helped a great deal. He may have experienced the therapist during his treatment as passing his tests and offering him pro-plan interpretations, and thus as disagreeing with his pathogenic beliefs and expressing sympathy toward his goals. The patient at the beginning of therapy may conjecture that his pathogenic beliefs are false and that his goals are reasonable. However, at the end of therapy—after he experiences the therapist as disagreeing with his beliefs and as sympathetic to his goals—he may, while not demonstrating much more insight than at the beginning, have much more conviction about this insight.

At this point the reader may wonder how to reconcile our finding—that the patient who is given a series of pro-plan interpretations demonstrates an immediate increase in experiencing and insight after each interpretation—with our finding that his total insight per hour is decreasing in the descending part of the parabolic curve. Our explanation of this is as follows: While the patient is testing the therapist, he feels anxious and defensive. Immediately after a pro-plan interpretation that passes his test, the patient feels slightly more secure. He also feels a small but measurable sense of relief, and shows a small but measurable increase in insight. However, he may retain this relief only briefly. Rather than retaining it, he uses his greater security with the therapist to test the therapist more vigorously than before. This behavior may be compared to that of a man who is working hard to accomplish an important task, and who discovers that he has inherited a moderate amount of money. He immediately feels relieved and more secure; however, rather than retaining his sense of relief and security, he uses his new capital to work harder than ever to achieve his goals. Similarly, the patient works by testing. When the therapist's good interpretations pass his tests, he may feel more secure and work harder than ever by testing more vigorously.

This study supports our concepts that the patient tests the therapist throughout therapy, and that he does so according to a plan. The idea that the patient is following an unconscious plan explains our finding that a graph of his insight follows a parabolic curve that fits the length of the therapy plus the evaluation interviews. The patient, as discussed above, unconsciously controls his level of testing in order to obtain maximum help from the therapist.

Our findings should be of theoretical interest to all therapists, but should be especially useful to therapists who practice brief time-limited psychotherapy. As the findings indicate, the therapist may expect to learn about the patient's pathogenic beliefs and goals at the beginning of therapy. Then, if the patient appears to be losing insight during the first half or more of the therapy, the therapist need not become disheartened. The patient's loss of insight may be a sign not that the therapist is on the wrong track, but rather that the therapist is passing the patient's tests and so providing the patient with the security that enables him to test more vigorously.

Proposition VI
   The analytic patient may make steady progress, with ups and downs throughout the course of his treatment.

The sixth proposition was tested and supported in two studies of the analysis of Mrs. C. These studies showed that Mrs. C. worked steadily throughout her treatment at the task of disconfirming her pathogenic beliefs. At the beginning of treatment, she was weighed down by the pathogenic beliefs that she was responsible for the happiness of her parents and siblings; that in order not to challenge her parents, she should be helpless and timid; that she should not brag; and that since her parents could not express affection directly, she should not do so either. During her analysis she gradually succeeded in disconfirming these beliefs. She became progressively bolder, more able to express affection, more in control of herself, more able to brag, and more aware of her fear of hurting others.

In our first study (Shilkret, Isaacs, Drucker, & Curtis 1986), we measured changes during the first 100 sessions of Mrs. C.'s analysis in the degree to which Mrs. C. was aware of two of her pathogenic beliefs: that she was responsible for the happiness of others, and that she had the omnipotent power to hurt them. Shilkret's method was straightforward. She first had judges locate in the transcripts of the first 100 sessions of Mrs. C.'s analysis all speech segments containing references to these pathogenic beliefs. She then presented these segments in random order to independent judges, who rated them in accordance with a scale defining five levels of the patient's awareness of these beliefs. At the lowest level, Mrs. C. was unaware of these beliefs; at the highest level, she was aware of the beliefs and beginning to realize that they were irrational. The findings indicated that during the first 100 sessions of Mrs. C.'s analysis she worked steadily to disconfirm her belief in her omnipotent responsibility for others and in her power to hurt them. She became progressively more aware of these beliefs, and she began to realize that they were irrational. She also became more comfortable in experiencing real power (as opposed to magical omnipotence) in her relations with others.

A separate study carried out by Shilkret, Isaacs, Drucker, and Curtis (1986) demonstrated that Mrs. C. did the work described above largely unaided by analytic interpretation. Mrs. C.'s analyst (as he informed us after Mrs. C. had terminated treatment with him) did not consider Mrs. C.'s unconscious feelings of guilt and omnipotence to be an important part of her psychopathology. Nor did he interpret these to her during the sessions studied by Shilkret, except occasionally in response to her own statements that she felt either guilt or an omnipotent sense of responsibility. In these interpretations the therapist did nothing more than agree with Mrs. C's own assessments of herself.

The second study (Ransohoff, Drucker, & Sampson, 1987) was modeled after Shilkret's. It used five scales to measure Mrs. C.'s progress in disconfirming her pathogenic beliefs over the 1,114 sessions of her analysis. These scales were designed to measure Mrs. C.'s progress in recovering insights and in becoming less inhibited. In applying these scales, the investigators used a sampling technique. They applied the scales to 7 sequences of 12 sessions each, spaced relatively evenly throughout the entire treatment; thus they applied the scales to 84 sessions.

The five scales measured Mrs. C.'s capacity (1) to be fond of others, (2) to be bold, (3) to be aware of her fear of hurting others, (4) to brag, and (5) to be aware of her sense of responsibility toward others. The research was done very much as in the first study. The findings showed that throughout her analysis Mrs. C. made progress along each scale. However, though all changes were in the predicted direction, only the changes in her capacity to be bold and to feel affection were statistically significant.

The above-cited findings throw light on the process by which a patient changes his pathogenic beliefs. In most instances he works slowly over a long period of time to convince himself that the beliefs are false. He works both by using the therapist's interpretations, and by having new experience with the therapist. These findings support the usefulness of long-term therapy.

The idea that throughout an analysis the patient progressively disconfirms his pathogenic beliefs, and by doing so both gains confidence in the analyst and increases his control over his unconscious mental life, readily explains the stages of an analysis that Freud conceptualized in terms of the formation and resolution of the transference neurosis. The stage conceptualized by Freud as the formation of the transference neurosis comes about as the patient, during the first part of his analysis, begins to gain confidence in the analyst and to realize that his pathogenic beliefs are false, so that he gains greater control over his unconscious mental life. He may then unconsciously decide that he can safely both (1) love the therapist more than before, and (2) test his pathogenic beliefs more vigorously and dramatically than before by offering the therapist powerful transference tests, in the hope of obtaining even more evidence that his beliefs are false and maladaptive.

The stage of therapy conceptualized by Freud as the resolution of the transference neurosis comes about as a consequence of the patient's gaining considerably more conviction that his pathogenic beliefs are false and maladaptive, and thus of acquiring considerably greater control over his unconscious mental life and considerably more confidence in the analyst. At this stage the patient has less need to test his pathogenic beliefs vigorously, and he can use his better control over his mental life to behave appropriately in relation to the analyst and to others. As the patient stops testing his pathogenic beliefs vigorously, he appears to have resolved his transference neurosis.

Relationship of the Present Theory to Freud's 1911–1915 Theory and to His Late Theories

In this chapter I compare the theories of the mind and technique proposed here to both Freud's 1911–1915 theory and his late theories.[1] I show that my ideas contrast sharply with those of the 1911–1915 theory, but are highly compatible with concepts that Freud developed in his late writings as part of his ego psychology. I wish to emphasize the differences between my views and those of the 1911–1915 theory, because despite Freud's late theorizing, the early theory remains extremely influential (Lipton, 1967; Coltrera & Ross, 1967; Kanzer & Blum, 1967). Most present-day theories contain important elements of the 1911–1915 theory. They make use of Freud's late ideas only to the extent that these ideas may be fitted into the 1911–1915 theory without basically changing it.

For example, in their clinical thinking few therapists rely on the concepts of unconscious cognition and unconscious control that Freud developed in his late writings. Moreover, most present-day theorists, like Freud in the 1911–1915 theory, consider formulations in terms of powerful unconscious motiva-

[1] For a more detailed discussion of this topic, see Weiss et al. (1986), Chapter 2.

tions such as greed, lust and envy to be basic. In this assumption, the present theory contrasts sharply with the 1911–1915 theory, for I assume that the powerful motivations described above are held in place by unconscious (pathogenic) beliefs.

In his early work Freud based his concepts of the mind on what may be described as the "automatic-functioning hypothesis" (AFH). He assumed that the unconscious mind consists of powerful psychic forces—namely, impulses and defenses—that are regulated "automatically" (Freud, 1900, p. 600; 1905, p. 266) by the pleasure principle. Such regulation is beyond the patient's control and does not take account of his thoughts, beliefs or assessments of current reality. The impulses are close to instinct, and relatively untouched by reality, and they seek immediate gratification. The defenses oppose their coming forth. The interactions of the impulses and defenses are dynamic: Two equal and opposite forces may nullify each other, a strong force may overwhelm a weak one; or two tangential forces may give rise to compromise behavior that satisfies both. From the dynamic interactions of the impulses and defenses are derived almost all of the phenomena of psychic life (Freud, 1926b, p. 265).

THE DEVELOPMENT OF THE
HIGHER-MENTAL-FUNCTIONING HYPOTHESIS

Over a period of years—especially between 1920 and 1940, during which time he developed his ego psychology—Freud changed his early views about unconscious mental functioning. He based parts of his ego psychology on the assumption that a person may do unconsciously many of the same kinds of things that he does consciously. This assumption, which I have called the "higher mental functioning hypothesis" (HMFH), is the basis of the theory that is the subject of this book.

Freud presented the AFH most completely and adhered to it most fully in *The Interpretation of Dreams* (1900). However, even there he made use of a key idea of the HMFH—namely, the unconscious regulation of repression by the criteria of danger and safety. According to this idea, a person may unconsciously decide whether he may safely experience a previously repressed mental content, and then, on the basis of this decision, regulate its access to consciousness. If he unconsciously decides that he may safely experience the content, he may lift the repressions opposing its emergence and bring it forth. Freud (1900, pp. 567–568) used this idea to explain the expression in dreams of impulses that are repressed in waking life. He assumed that the censor (in his later writings, the ego) regulates impulse expression by the criteria of danger and safety. The censor may permit repressed impulses to be expressed in dreams, because the dreamer's power of motility has been shut down while he is asleep. Since the dreamer cannot act on his impulses, he may safely become conscious of them.

Freud never completely gave up the idea of automatic regulation by the pleasure principle. However, as he developed his ego psychology (Freud, 1923, 1926a, 1940a), he progressively limited the role of unconscious automatic regulation. He introduced unconscious motives that are not pleasure-seeking; that seek long-term rather than immediate goals; and that are regulated not automatically by the pleasure principle, but by higher mental functions.

Freud based these modifications of his theory on clinical observation. He changed his early views about the importance of pleasure seeking in unconscious mental life when he observed that patients unconsciously repeat, both in their dreams and in relation to the analyst, traumatic experiences that are not and never were pleasurable (1920, p. 24); he changed his views about the scope of the pleasure principle when he observed the great part played by guilt and masochism in mental life (1937, p. 242).

Freud was also induced to alter his early views about unconscious automatic functioning by his growing conviction about the importance of the castration complex in the psychopathology of the male. Castration anxiety is not pleasurable, and it does not arise automatically but from a belief that is derived from experience by normal processes of inference (1940b, p. 277). Nor does it arise in fantasy as Freud defined the concept; fantasy, according to Freud, is wishful and exempt from reality testing (1911, p. 222). However, the belief in castration is not wishful, and rather than leading away from reality, it is about reality (1926a, p. 108). Freud repeatedly described castration anxiety as arising not from a fantasy but from a belief (see 1940b, p. 277).

The idea that a person may be guided unconsciously by deeply repressed beliefs made it necessary for Freud to postulate an executive agency, the ego, part of which may be deeply repressed. Freud introduced this agency in *The Ego and the Id* (1923). In the same work he introduced another agency, the superego (a part of the ego), which may be deeply repressed and which operates by higher mental functions (pp. 26–27). Moreover, the superego may give rise to motives that are not necessarily pleasurable and that may be intensely painful.

In *Inhibitions, Symptoms, and Anxiety* (1926a) Freud wrote explicitly that the ego may unconsciously regulate behavior by thought (rather than by automatic processes). He developed this idea still further in the New Introductory Lectures on Psycho-Analysis (1933, pp. 89–90) and in *An Outline of Psycho-Analysis* (1940a, p. 199). In the latter, Freud wrote:

> Its [the ego's] constructive function consists of interpolating, between the demand made by an instinct and the action that satisfies it, the activity of thought which, after taking its bearings in the present and assessing earlier experiences, endeavors by means of experimental actions to calculate the consequences of the courses of action proposed. In this way the ego comes to a decision on whether the attempt to obtain satisfaction is to be carried out or postponed, or whether it may be necessary for the demand by the instinct to be suppressed altogether as being dangerous. (Here we have the *reality principle*.) Just as the id is directed exclusively to obtaining pleasure, so the ego is governed by considerations of safety. The ego has set itself the task of self-preservation which the id appears to neglect. (1940a, p. 199)

In this passage Freud assumed that a person is powerfully motivated unconsciously to assess his reality. He attempts to determine the dangers his reality presents, in order to decide whether to carry out a proposed course of action, to delay carrying it out, or to suppress it. The person (or his ego), in making this decision, thinks unconsciously about the proposed action. He considers the present situation and compares it with past experiences, in order to gauge the consequences of performing the action. He also makes use unconsciously of "experimental actions"—that is, tests of the environment—as part of his effort to determine whether he can safely perform the action.

In his ego psychology, Freud described two additional unconscious mental processes that run counter to the AFH and that pertain to the theory of technique that is the subject of this book. The first, which Freud introduced tentatively in *Beyond the Pleasure Principle* (1920), is an unconscious wish for mastery. Freud suggested that a patient may unconsciously repeat traumatic experiences not for gratification, but in order to master them, just as children in play repeat traumatic experiences in order to master them (p. 35). In *Analysis Terminable and Interminable* (1937) Freud developed this concept further by strongly implying that the patient works unconsciously with the analyst to solve his problems. He wrote that "the analytic situation consists in our allying ourselves with the ego of the person under treatment, in order to subdue portions of his id that are uncontrolled—that is to say, to include them in the synthesis of his ego" (p. 235). In the Outline (1940a), Freud developed these concepts still further by assigning the ego "the task of self-preservation" (p. 199), and by assuming that the ego carries out this task by gaining control of the demands of the instincts (p. 146) and by regulating behavior by the criteria of danger and safety (p. 199).

The other unconscious process that Freud introduced in his ego psychology and that runs counter to the AFH is the process of unconscious identification (1923, pp. 29–30). Such identification, Freud wrote, is important for the development of both the ego and the superego. The concept of identification contradicts the AFH, in that it points to the importance of experience in the development of motivation. Moreover, as noted above, the concept of the superego emphasizes the importance of motives that are not impulses seeking immediate gratification, but rather are persistent and may be painful.

In each of the ideas of his ego psychology outlined above,

Freud postulated an unconscious mental process that is similar to a familiar conscious mental process. According to these ideas, a person may unconsciously think, decide, and plan. In making his plans, he may rely on unconscious beliefs about reality and morality. He may unconsciously assess his current reality. He may learn by identifying with others. He may be strongly motivated unconsciously to solve his problems, and in therapy he may work with the therapist to do this.

FREUD'S LATE THEORY LED TO NEW CONCEPTUALIZATIONS OF CLINICAL PHENOMENA

Freud's late theory, with its ideas about unconscious cognition, ego interests, anxiety, guilt, restitution, and identification, led to numerous new conceptualizations of clinical phenomena. It permitted the clinician to discriminate between behaviors that in the early theory are all assumed to express primary impulses. Thus behaviors that express a primary impulse, according to the early theory, may arise in the ego and superego, according to the late theory.

For example, behavior that arises in the superego may be conceptualized not as expressing the pursuit of gratification, but as expressing a wish to atone, to sacrifice, or to be punished. Thus a patient's sexual attachment to a love object, which in Freud's early theory is seen as the expression of a primary impulse seeking gratification, may be understood according to the late theory as motivated by a wish to restore the love object. For example, a patient who suffers from an exaggerated sense of responsibility for the therapist and who believes he has hurt him may attempt by loving him to restore him. Such a patient is seeking not gratification but relief of guilt. Moreover, his behavior is regulated not automatically but by beliefs—namely, by his belief in his responsibility for the therapist, and by his belief in the power of his love to restore the therapist. Nor in this instance is the patient's love for the therapist a defense, as conceptualized in the early theory. Unlike the defenses of the early theory, it is not regulated automatically by the pleasure principle, nor is it intended to ward off infantile gratification. Rather, it is intended to reassure against guilt and worry.

Another example of behavior that arises in the superego is that of a patient who is self-destructive in order to protect himself against Oedipal guilt. For example, a patient may retain his childish temper tantrums so as to prevent himself from surpassing his father, whose own temper tantrums prevented him from being happily married. In this instance, the patient's temper is not the direct expression of a primary affect or impulse, nor is it regulated automatically. Instead, it is regulated by the patient's belief that if he surpasses his father and so permits himself marital happiness, he will risk hurting his father or being punished by him.

Behavior that in Freud's early theory is conceptualized as the expression of a primary sadistic impulse may be conceptualized in the late theory as arising in the ego; it may express the ego defense of identification with the aggressor (A. Freud, 1936). For example, a patient may be sadistic to the analyst, as a parent was to him. This concept marks an advance over the early theory, which assumes that defenses simply ward off impulses seeking gratification. The defense of identification with the aggressor is assumed to ward off not an impulse seeking gratification, but anxiety or humiliation arising from trauma.

Another example is the patient who uses a fetish to arouse himself sexually. In the early theory, such behavior is conceptualized as expressing the patient's primary attachment to the fetish. In the late theory, it may be conceptualized as reassuring the patient against castration anxiety arising from his belief in castration as a punishment. Here, too, the patient's behavior is mediated not automatically by the pleasure principle, but in accordance with a belief acquired by the patient in the traumas of childhood.

Also according to the late theory, a person may do things out of ego interests and not simply as the expression of a defense, an impulse, or a compromise between these. He may, in deciding unconsciously upon a goal, take into account his various impulses, his conscience, and his opportunities. Then, having set the goal, he may work to realize it.

SOME IMPLICATIONS OF FREUD'S LATE THEORY FOR TECHNIQUE

As many analysts have pointed out, ego psychology has not greatly influenced the psychoanalytic theory of technique (Lipton, 1967; Coltrera & Ross, 1967; Kanzer & Blum, 1967), because the theory of technique was evolved by Freud before he developed his ego psychology and so was cast largely in the mold of the AFH. Freud's powerful and systematic presentation in the *Papers on Technique* (1911–1915) has remained the basis for much psychoanalytic thinking about technique up to the present time.

Most current versions of the psychoanalytic theory of technique retain many of the fundamental features of the 1911–1915 theory. Technical ideas based on the HMFH have been added onto an existing theory without any organic change in the theory. Nor have the technical applications of the HMFH been systematically spelled out. In contrast to most current versions of the psychoanalytic theory of technique, the theory that is the subject of this book is built from the ground up on the concepts of the HMFH.

Although the psychoanalytic theory of technique has resisted influence by ego psychology, it has nonetheless been somewhat altered by it. Thus present-day psychoanalytic theories differ from the 1911–1915 theory in their answers to such questions as "What are the patient's tasks?" "How does the patient work in treatment?" and "How does the analyst help the patient?"

The Patient's Tasks

The patient's tasks, as originally conceptualized by Freud, are to free himself from his attachment to certain infantile aims and objects, and to redirect the freed energy to more mature aims and to new objects. In Freud's original formulations, the accomplishment of these tasks was assumed, in theory if not in practice, to be relatively simple and direct: The patient is helped by the analyst's interpretations to become conscious of his infantile impulses, to gain control of them, and to redirect the libido contained in them along more mature lines. However, as the psychoanalytic theory of technique assimilated certain of Freud's late ideas, the patient's tasks came to be seen as more complex than originally formulated. They came to be seen as requiring the accomplishment of a number of subsidiary tasks, none of which were conceivable in the early theory.

For example, the new concepts about unconscious identification gave rise to the technical idea that the patient, to accomplish his goals, may have to undo certain pathological identifications. For another example, the new concepts about the superego that Freud developed in *The Ego and the Id* (1923) gave rise to the technical idea that the patient may have to develop a milder superego. Also, the new concepts that Freud put forth about the development of castration anxiety and its role in psychopathology (1926a) gave rise to the technical ideas that the patient may have to change a belief (the belief in castration), and overcome the effects of certain childhood traumas.

How the Patient Works

Freud's early formulations about how the patient works in treatment were relatively simple. In these formulations Freud assumed that the patient's work is mainly conscious. He works out of love for the analyst, by free-associating and by understanding and assimilating the insights that the analyst conveys to him through interpretation. However, as Freud developed new ideas about the mind, he created a more complex view of how the patient may work. For example, Freud's concept of unconscious identification as developed in *The Ego and the Id* (1923) gave rise to the idea that the patient may work unconsciously or perhaps preconsciously by making temporary identifications with the analyst (Gitelson, 1962; Loewenstein, 1954). Thus he may benefit by identifying with the analyst's patience, neutrality, and matter-of-fact approach, and in addition with the analyst's more benign superego (Strachey, 1934).

Freud's new ideas about the importance of unconscious guilt and unconscious cognition in mental life stimulated certain analysts to focus on the importance of guilt in the development and maintenance of psychopathology. For example, Modell (1965, 1971) has written about the part played by survivor guilt and separation guilt in the lives of many patients. These forms of guilt, which Modell considers widespread or perhaps universal, may impede a patient in the pursuit of normal goals. Moreover, Modell has implied that such guilt is based on beliefs (1965, p. 330; 1971, p. 339), and that the patient, in order to overcome such guilt, must change these beliefs.

Freud's new ideas about the part played by an unconscious pathogenic belief (i.e., the belief in castration) in the development and maintenance of psychopathology suggested to some analysts that the patient may work with the analyst by acquiring new experiences with him. The reasoning behind this suggestion is straightforward: If, as Freud assumed in *Inhibitions, Symptoms and Anxiety* (1926a), a patient suffers from a pathogenic belief acquired in experience, he may be helped by fresh experiences to change this belief. That Freud was concerned with how the patient is affected by his experiences with the analyst is suggested by certain passages scattered throughout his late works. A good example is the following, in which Freud warned the analyst not to impose his values on the patient. Freud wrote that if the analyst does this, "He [the analyst] will only be repeating a mistake of the parents who crushed their child's independence by their influence, and he will only be replacing the patient's earlier dependence by a new one" (1940a, p. 175). This statement indicates that the therapist may help the patient, or at least not harm him, by offering him experiences different from his childhood experiences with his parents.

The role of the patient's experiences with the analyst was emphasized by Anna Freud (1959), who stated that the patient extracts from his relationship to the analyst the experiences he needs in order to do his work. Also, Alexander and French (1946, pp. 20–24) wrote that the patient may benefit from certain "corrective emotional experiences." Rangell (1981b), years later, agreed with Alexander and French that the patient may benefit from corrective emotional experiences, but suggested that the patient benefits more from what the analyst does not do than from what he does.

Rangell, who bases much of his theorizing on Freud's late

ideas (such as the ideas that the patient unconsciously thinks, decides, and is guided by maladaptive beliefs), also assumes that the patient may actively seek from the analyst the experiences he needs to disconfirm his maladaptive beliefs and to overcome the anxiety stemming from them. The patient, according to Rangell (1969a, 1969b), may seek such experiences unconsciously by testing the analyst. Dewald (1976, 1978) has likewise pointed to the patient's unconscious testing of the analyst. Kohut (1984) has assumed that the patient, through new experiences with the analyst, may correct and begin to overcome certain developmental deficits.

Freud stimulated psychoanalytic thinking by his idea that the patient may work unconsciously to master his problems (1920, pp. 32, 35), and also by the related idea that the patient may develop a therapeutic alliance with the analyst in order to subdue certain uncontrolled parts of the id (*Analysis Terminable and Interminable*, 1937, p. 235). Freud's concept of the therapeutic alliance was subsequently developed by several analysts, including Greenson (1965, 1967) and Zetzel and Meissner (1973). Kris (1950, 1951, 1956a, 1956b) assumed that the patient, in working to master his problems, may exert control over his repressions. He may lift his defenses and bring forth warded-off memories as part of his working to master his unconscious mental life. Also, Loewenstein (1954) and Loewald (1960) both assumed that the patient may bring forth warded-off transferences in order to master them.

Greenson (1967) assumed that in analysis the patient may repeat frightening experiences in order to master them. In some of his case discussions, he wrote that the patient brought forth new material when he unconsciously considered it safe to do so. He therefore implied that the patient unconsciously may use thought to assess his current reality, and that he may act on such assessments.

How the Analyst May Help the Patient

Freud's early ideas about what the analyst does are relatively simple, in concept if not in practice. The analyst enjoins the patient to free-associate. He maintains an impersonal, investigatory attitude toward the patient, and he uses the patient's associations to interpret the unconscious impulses, affects, and defenses that underlie his symptoms and character problems.

These technical ideas are still widely accepted. However, new concepts about the analyst's task were stimulated by Freud's ego psychology. The idea that the patient may regulate his repressions by the criteria of danger and safety inspired Bernfeld (1941) to imply strongly that the therapist should help the patient to feel safe with him. The ideas that the patient should develop a therapeutic alliance and an observing ego suggested to Greenson (1967) that the analyst should help the patient to develop these. The idea that the patient may work by testing the analyst (Freud, 1940a, p. 199; Rangell, 1969a, 1969b) implied that the analyst should understand the patient's tests and pass them.

Freud's early ideas about the nature of unconscious motivation also had important implications for how the analyst can help the patient. In his early theorizing, Freud assumed that repressed motivations are all the same kinds of thing—namely, impulses seeking immediate gratification and defenses opposing the impulses' coming forth. They are psychic forces regulated by the pleasure principle, beyond the patient's control and unorganized by thought, belief, or plan. Moreover all of these psychic forces are primary, and all are on the same level in the psychic hierarchy. The idea that they are all on the same level is shown by the assumption that they are additive.

These formulations gave rise to the idea that the analyst should be impartial to the impulses. That is, he should not favor one impulse over another, but should impartially deny each impulse its gratification. In the early theory, impartiality is by implication an aspect of neutrality. An analyst who is impartial to all motivations is, by definition, also neutral.

In Freud's late theorizing, unconscious motivation includes not only primary impulses seeking gratification, but motives stemming from the unconscious parts of the ego and superego, and serving a variety of purposes and functions. These new concepts changed earlier ideas about how the analyst should position himself relative to the patient's unconscious motives. For example, Anna Freud's recommendation (1936) that the analyst position himself equally distant from the ego, superego, and id indicated a change from the early view, which did not require the analyst in positioning himself to consider any unconscious motivations except primary impulses. Anna Freud's later recommendation (1959), that the analyst frustrate the drives but support the ego in its attempts at mastery, explicitly changed the earlier idea that the analyst be impartial to all unconscious motivations. Thus it altered the early concept of neutrality.

CHAPTER 10

A Comparison of the Present Theory with Other Current Theories

The present theory, with its emphasis on the patient's wish to master his problems, is related to the views of Loewald (1960) and Settlage (personal communication, 1989) in assuming that the patient is motivated in therapy to complete certain developmental tasks. The present theory is also an object relations theory in that it assumes (as do many other theories today), that the patient develops his problems in relation to his first objects, his parents and siblings, and that he may resolve his problems in relation to another object, the therapist (Sullivan, 1940; Winnicott, 1965; Lichtenberg, 1983a, 1983b; Stolorow & Lachmann, 1984–1985; Kernberg, 1977, 1987; Thoma & Kachele, 1992).

The present theory is related to self psychology (Kohut, 1959, 1971, 1984), which is also an object relations theory. Both theories emphasize that the patient's problems arise in his early experiences with his parents, and that the patient benefits from new experiences with the therapist. Neither theory subscribes to the idea that the therapist should be neutral and impersonal. Neither theory prohibits warmth or empathy. Moreover, in some (but certainly not all), instances, the technical recommendations prescribed by self psychology and those prescribed by the present theory are compatible: Behavior that, according to self psychology, offers the patient the empathy he needs may, according to the present theory, pass the patient's tests.

However, there are many differences between these two theories, several of which I indicate here. Self psychology emphasizes the great part played in psychopathology by shame and humiliation arising in early childhood in relationships with unempathic parents. The present theory agrees that shame and humiliation are important in psychopathology, but adds that these affect states are maintained partly for moral reasons, and thus by unconscious guilt. In the present formulation, the child who develops a sense of shame in relation to unempathic and derisive parents comes to believe that he should be ashamed. He regards his parents as absolute authorities on reality and morality, and so believes that the ways they treat him are justified on both real and moral grounds. Later in life, if he resists feeling ashamed, he may develop guilt to his parents. He may experience his lack of shame as expressing disloyalty. Alternatively, he may become sad, for by being disloyal to his parents he may be breaking his ties to them.

From the point of view of the present theory, self psychology underestimates the importance for the development of psychopathology of various forms of guilt, including survivor guilt, separation guilt, and guilt arising from an exaggerated sense of responsibility for others. For this reason, the self psychologist may not discriminate clearly between the patient who suffers primarily from narcissistic wounds and so requires the nurturing prescribed by self psychology, and the patient who behaves as though he is in need of nurturing in order not to reject the therapist, who he assumes is gratified by nurturing him. Moreover, a patient who infers from a symbiotic worried mother that he has no right to feel differently than she feels may want his therapist to demonstrate a capacity, not to empathize in the narrow sense, but to feel separate.

The present theory is also related to cognitive psychology (Beck, Rush, Shaw, & Emery, 1979; Persons, 1989). Both theories assume that the patient suffers from maladaptive beliefs, and that psychotherapy is a process in which the patient is helped by the therapist to change these beliefs. The two theories overlap as regards the kinds of beliefs with which they are concerned. However, the present theory, more than cognitive psychology, assumes that each patient is concerned with just a few broad beliefs that he acquired in early childhood, and that reflect the concerns of the infant or young child in his relations to his parents.

The two theories also differ as to how the patient may be helped by the therapist to change his maladaptive beliefs. According to the cognitive psychologist, such beliefs may be outside the patient's awareness. The therapist uses discussion and questioning to focus the patient's attention on the beliefs and to help the patient to realize that the beliefs are false and maladaptive. The present theory assumes that the beliefs may be repressed and unconscious. The therapist helps the patient to become conscious of the beliefs and to change them not only by interpretation, but by passing the patient's tests. In contrast to cognitive therapy the present theory assumes that the therapist may sometimes help the patient to change his pathogenic beliefs without use of interpretation, discussion, or questioning. He may help the patient simply by passing his tests.

The present theory agrees with Alexander and French (1946) about the benefits of a corrective emotional experience. Both theories advocate a case-specific approach, and both agree that the patient may be helped by his relationship with the therapist. However, the present theory, more than the theory of Alexander and French, puts the value of the corrective emotional experience in a theoretical context in which it makes sense. It does not make sense in the context of Freud's 1911–1915 theory, for in this theory the unconscious mind does not contain pathogenic beliefs that may be changed by new experiences. It does make sense in the context of the present theory, for this theory assumes that the patient suffers from pathogenic beliefs, and therefore that he may benefit from experiences that run counter to these beliefs.

In contrast to the theory of Alexander and French, the present theory offers a precise definition of the kinds of experience from which the patient may benefit. These are experiences that the patient himself is seeking by his testing of his pathogenic beliefs in relation to the therapist. In addition, the present theory differs from that of Alexander and French in that it offers the therapist a means of judging whether he is on the right track. If over a period of time the therapist passes the patient's tests, the patient will show improvement. If over a period of time he fails the patient's tests, the patient will be set back or reach an impasse.

The theory proposed here finds support in developmental psychology. For example, its emphasis on the higher-mental-functioning hypothesis and on the adaptive point of view are supported by the infant research of Stern (1985) and others (Brazelton & Yogman, 1989; Emde, 1989). As I have discussed in Chapter 2, Stern has demonstrated that the infant is power-fully motivated to adapt to his interpersonal world. In working to do so, the infant makes use of his higher mental functions; for example, he makes and tests hypotheses about how he may affect his mother and how she may react to him.

The present theory also encompasses the common-sense ways in which one person may help another. It assumes that in certain circumstances (depending on the patient's pathogenic beliefs) the therapist may help the patient by offering him en-couragement or reassurance, or by confronting him with his self-destructive behavior, or by using his authority to protect the patient from danger.

Unlike most current psychoanalytic theories, the present theory assumes that the patient's central organizing motive is to adapt to his interpersonal world. In its emphasis on adapta-tion, the present theory is in agreement with the theory of John Bowlby (1969). This emphasis contrasts with that of the 1911–1915 theory, which scarcely recognizes a wish for adaptation. In addition, the early theory of the mind on which Freud built the 1911–1915 theory of technique scarcely acknowledges the role of experience in development, except to affirm that the infant is forced by the exigencies of life to relinquish halluci-natory wish fulfillment and to seek gratification in the external world (Freud, 1900).

In his late works Freud wrote, mainly in brief theoretical passages, about the importance of the task of adaptation. For example, in *An Outline of Psycho-Analysis* (1940a), he wrote that a person is motivated by the wish to preserve himself (p. 199), and that in doing this he tests reality (p. 199), regulates his behavior by the criteria of safety and danger (p. 199), and strives to gain control of the demands of the instincts (p. 144).

After Freud, other theoreticians—for instance, Hartmann (1956a, 1956b)—have written about the person's wish to adapt to reality. However neither Hartmann nor other theoreticians have assumed that the wish to adapt is the patient's central organizing motive. Moreover, though the importance of the wish to adapt has been acknowledged in theory, it has scarcely affected the thinking of many clinicians, who continue to perceive their patients as motivated primarily by sexual and aggressive impulses and not by the wish to adapt to their worlds. For example, today many analysts consider explanations in terms of lust, greed, envy, jealousy, rage, hatred, and so forth to be primary. In their views, once a therapist demonstrates that a motive of this kind underlies certain behavior, he has gone as far as he can in explaining this behavior. If, as I assume, lust, greed, envy, jealousy, hatred and so forth are held in place by pathogenic beliefs, then the "daemonic" in human life is not sustained primarily by instinct. However, it may be sustained by conscience. For example, as reported in Chapter 2, a female patient developed an overwhelming, maladaptive sexual interest in a male acquaintance as a consequence of survivor guilt about her mother. She had been proud of her control over her sexuality, but she developed a feeling of being overwhelmed by her sexuality as a consequence of her guilt about being a better person than her mother, who had no such control. As this patient was helped by the therapist to understand that her overwhelming sexual interest arose in guilt, she re-established control over it.

My technical approach is distinctive in its recommendation that throughout therapy the therapist should develop as comprehensive a picture of the patient and his problems as he can derive from his current knowledge of the patient. From the beginning of therapy, the therapist attempts to formulate the patient's pathogenic beliefs, goals, and plans, and the origins of these in the patient's childhood. He expands and refines these formulations as he learns more about the patient in the course of therapy. A comprehensive formulation may enable the therapist to see a remarkable continuity in the patient's diverse and shifting affects, impulses, and behaviors; it may thus guide the therapist in his attempts to help the patient to disprove his pathogenic beliefs and to pursue his goals.

A good plan formulation is crucial, for the only technical rule broad enough to offer the therapist optimal guidance in his work with the patient is this: "Infer the patient's pathogenic beliefs and goals, and help the patient to disprove these beliefs and to pursue these goals." No group of technical rules, no matter how subtle—including such rules as "Maintain an atmosphere of abstinence," or "Demonstrate your empathy or your appreciation of the patient's perspective," or "Investigate the resistances behind the patient's changes of topic"—is broad enough to encompass the various pathogenic beliefs from which a patient suffers, and the various ways he may test these beliefs with his therapist.

The therapist who bases his technique on such rules may assume that he is analyzing a resistance or frustrating a repressed impulse. However, from the patient's point of view, the therapist is demonstrating either sympathy with the patient's goals, opposition to them, or indifference to them. The patient is always concerned with assuring himself that the therapist disagrees with his pathogenic beliefs and is in sympathy with his goals. Regardless of the therapist's intentions, this is what the patient is interested in, and this is what he observes and reacts to.

The therapist shows the patient that throughout therapy he is working to disprove just a few pathogenic beliefs and pursue just a few goals. Also, he helps the patient to understand how his pathogenic beliefs arose in early childhood from real experiences with his parents and from his reasonable efforts to maintain his ties to them. He thereby may help the patient to overcome the feeling that he is inherently different, defective, or bad. The patient comes to realize that another child, confronted with a reality similar to his, might have developed similar pathogenic beliefs. Thus the therapist should help the patient to understand that the development of his pathogenic beliefs and symptoms was not a mysterious process, but an effort at adaptation to his reality.

List of Case References
(in Order of Appearance in Text)

CHAPTER 1

Sylvia G.
Andrea M.

CHAPTER 2

Alex N.
Talia S.
Mrs. C.
Marla L.
Randall D.
Ruth Z.

CHAPTER 3

Roberta P.
Willa A.
Geoffrey B.
Timothy E.
Lowell A.
Karen B.
Teresa K.

CHAPTER 4

Harriet A.
Stuart C.
Kenneth Y.
Leonard C.
Zora T.

Janice D.
Francine A.
Kirsten C.

CHAPTER 5

William W.
Arthur D.
Terry W.
Valerie T.
Nancy C.
Darlene S.
Margaret M.
Thomas Y.
Stephan X.
Lisa O.
Gina H.
Felice M.
Gloria S.
Walter A.
Lyle K.
Donald G.
Davis F.
Allan C.

CHAPTER 6

Thomas C. (continued)
Esther A.
Katherine A.

References

Alexander, F., & French, T. M. (1946). *Psychoanalytic therapy: Principles and application.* New York: Ronald Press.

Asch, S. (1976). Varieties of negative therapeutic reaction and problems of technique. *Journal of the American Psychoanalytic Association, 24,* 383–407.

Balson, P. (1975). *Dreams and fantasies as adaptive mechanisms in prisoners of war in Vietnam.* Unpublished manuscript written in consultation with M. Horowitz and E. Erikson. (On file at the San Francisco Psychoanalytic Institute)

Beck, A. T., Rush, A. J., Shaw, B. F., & Emery, G. (1979). *Cognitive therapy of depression.* New York: Guilford Press.

Beres, D. (1958). Certain aspects of superego functioning. *Psychoanalytic Study of the Child, 13,* 324–351.

Bernfeld, S. (1941). The facts of observation in psychoanalysis. *International Review of Psychoanalysis, 12*(3), 342–351.

Bibring, E. (1954). Psychoanalysis and the dynamic psychotherapies. *Journal of the American Psychoanalytic Association, 2*(1), 245–270.

Bowlby, J. (1969). *Attachment and loss: Vol 1. Attachment.* New York: Basic Books.

Brazelton, T. B., & Yogman, M. W. (Eds.). (1989). *Affective development in infancy.* Norwood, NJ: Ablex.

Broitman, J. (1985). Insight, the mind's eye: An exploration of three patients' processes of becoming insightful (Doctoral dissertation, Wright Institute Graduate School of Psychology). *Dissertation Abstracts International, 1985, 46*(8b). (University Microfilms No. 85-20,425)

Brown, S. (1985). *Treating the alcoholic: A developmental model of recovery.* New York: Wiley.

Brown, S. (1988). *Treating adult children of alcoholics: A developmental perspective.* New York: Wiley.

Bruner, J. S. (1977). Early social interaction and language acquisition. In H. R. Schaffer (Ed.), *Studies in mother–infant interaction*. London: Academic Press.

Bugas, J. (1986). Adaptive regression in the therapeutic change process (Doctoral dissertation, Pacific Graduate Schoolof Psychology). *Dissertation Abstracts International*, 1986, 47(7b), (University Microfilms No. 86-22,826)

Bush, M., & Gassner, S. (1986). The immediate effect of the analyst's termination interventions on the patient's resistance to termination. In J. Weiss, H. Sampson, & the Mount Zion Psychotherapy Research Group (Eds.), *The psychoanalytic process: Theory, clinical observation & empirical research*. (pp. 299–320). New York: Guilford Press.

Caston, J. (1986). The reliability of the diagnosis of the patient's unconscious plan. In J. Weiss, H. Sampson, & the Mount Zion Psychotherapy Research Group (Eds.), *The psychoanalytic process: Theory, clinical observation & empirical research*. (pp. 241–255). New York: Guilford Press.

Coltrera, J., & Ross, N. (1967). Freud's psychoanalytic technique—from beginnings to 1923. In B. Wolman (Ed.), *Psychoanalytic techniques: A handbook for the practicing psychoanalyst* (pp. 13–50). New York: Basic Books.

Curtis, J., & Silberschatz, G. (1986). Clinical implications of research on brief psychodynamic psychotherapy: I. Formulating the patient's problems and goals. *Psychoanalytic Psychology, 3*(1), 13–25.

Dahl, H. (1980, May). *New directions in affect theory*. Paper presented at the annual meeting of the American Psychoanalytic Association, New York.

Dahl, H., Kachele, H., & Thomä, H., (Eds.). (1988). *Psychoanalytic process research strategies*. Berlin: Springer-Verlag.

Davilla, L. (1992). *The immediate effects of therapist's interpretations on patient's plan progressiveness*. Unpublished doctoral dissertation, California School of Professional Psychology.

Dewald, P. A. (1976). Transference regression and real experience in the psychoanalytic process. *Psychoanalytic Quarterly, 45*(2), 213–230.

Dewald, P. A. (1978). The psychoanalytic process in adult patients. *Psychoanalytic Study of the Child, 33*, 323–332.

Edelstein, S. (1992). *Insight and psychotherapy outcome*. Unpublished doctoral dissertation, Wright Institute Graduate School of Psychology.

Emde, R.N. (1989). The infant's relationship experience: Developmental and affective aspects. In A.J. Sameroff & R.N. Emde (Eds.), *Relationship disturbances in early childhood: A developmental approach*. (pp. 33–51). New York: Basic Books.

Fretter, P. (1984). The immediate effects of transference interpretations on patients' progress in brief, psychodynamic psychotherapy (Doctoral dissertation, University of San Francisco). *Dissertation Abstracts International, 1985, 46*(6a). (University Microfilms No. 85-12,112)

Freud, A. (1936). *The ego and the mechanisms of defense.* New York: International Universities Press, 1946.

Freud, A. (1959). Paper presented at the San Francisco Psychoanalytic Institute.

Freud, S. (1900). The interpretation of dreams. *Standard Edition, 4,* 1–338; *5,* 339–627. London: Hogarth Press, 1953.

Freud, S. (1901). On dreams. *Standard Edition, 5,* 633–686. London: Hogarth Press, 1953.

Freud, S. (1905). On psychotherapy. *Standard Edition, 7,* 255–568. London: Hogarth Press, 1953.

Freud, S. (1911). Formulations on the two principles of mental functioning. *Standard Edition, 12,* 213–226. London: Hogarth Press, 1958.

Freud, S. (1911–1915). Papers on technique. *Standard Edition, 12,* 83–171. London: Hogarth Press, 1958.

Freud, S. (1920). Beyond the pleasure principle. *Standard Edition, 18,* 3–64. London: Hogarth Press, 1955.

Freud, S. (1923). The ego and the id. *Standard Edition, 19,* 3–66. London: Hogarth Press, 1961.

Freud, S. (1926a). Inhibitions, symptoms and anxiety. *Standard Edition, 20,* 77–175. London: Hogarth Press, 1959.

Freud, S. (1926b). Psycho-analysis. *Standard Edition, 20,* 259–270. London: Hogarth Press, 1959.

Freud, S. (1933). New introductory lectures on psycho-analysis. *Standard Edition, 22,* 3–182. London: Hogarth Press, 1964.

Freud, S. (1937). Analysis terminable and interminable. *Standard Edition, 23,* 209–253. London: Hogarth Press, 1964.

Freud, S. (1940a). An outline of psycho-analysis. *Standard Edition, 23,* 141–207. London: Hogarth Press, 1964.

Freud, S. (1940b). Splitting of the ego in the process of defense. *Standard Edition, 23,* 272–278. London: Hogarth Press, 1964.

Gassner, S. (1989). *The management and treatment of anxiety in psychotherapy.* Paper presented at the 15th Annual Midwinter Program in Continuing Education for Psychiatrists, University of California–Davis, 1989.

Gassner, S., Sampson, H., Weiss, J., & Brumer, S. (1982). The emergence of warded-off contents. *Psychoanalysis and Contemporary Thought, 5*(1), 55–75.

Gitelson, M. (1962). The curative factors in psychoanalysis. *International Journal of Psycho-Analysis, 43,* 194–205.

Gottschalk, L. A. (1974). The application of a method of content analysis to psychotherapy research. *American Journal of Psychotherapy, 28*(4), 488–499.

Greenberg, R., Katz, H., Schwartz, W., & Pearlman, C. (1992). Research based reconsideration of the psychoanalytic theory of dreaming. *Journal of the American Psychoanalytic Association, 40*(2), 531–550.

Greenson, R. R. (1965). The working alliance and the transference neurosis. *Psychoanalytic Quarterly, 34,* 155–181.

Greenson, R. R. (1967). *The technique and practice of psychoanalysis* (Vol. 1). New York: International Universities Press.

Hartmann, H. (1939). *Ego psychology and the problem of adaptation.* New York: International Universities Press, 1958.

Hartmann, H. (1956a). Notes on the reality principle. In H. Hartmann, *Essays on ego psychology* (pp. 241–267). New York: International Universities Press, 1964.

Hartmann, H. (1956b). The development of the ego concept in Freud's work. In H. Hartmann, *Essays on ego psychology.* (pp. 268–296). New York: International Universities Press, 1964.

Horowitz, M. J., (1991). *Person schemas and maladaptive interpersonal patterns.* Chicago: University of Chicago Press.

Horowitz, M. J., & Stinson, C. (1991). University of California, San Francisco, Center for the Study of Neuroses. Program on Conscious and Unconscious Mental Processes. In L. Beutler & M. Crago (Eds.), *Psychotherapy research: An international review in programmatic studies* (Chap. 13, pp. 107–114). Washington, DC: American Psychological Association.

Kanzer, M., & Blum, H. (1967). Classical psychoanalysis since 1939. In B. Wolman (Ed.), *Psychoanalytic Techniques: A Handbook for Practicing Psychoanalysts* (pp. 138–139). New York: Basic Books.

Kelly, T. (1989). *Do therapist's interventions matter?* Unpublished doctoral dissertation, New York University.

Kernberg, O. F. (1987). The structural diagnosis of borderline personality organization. In P. Hartocollis (Ed.), *Borderline personality disorders* (pp. 87–121). New York: International Universities Press.

Kernberg, O. F. (1987). Projection and projective identification: Developmental and clinical aspects. *Journal of the American Psychoanalytic Association, 35,* 795–819.

Klein, M. H., Mathieu, P. L., Gendlin, E. T., & Kiesler, D. J. (1970). *The Experiencing Scale: A research and training manual* (Vols. 1 and 2). Madison, WI: Psychiatric Institute, Bureau of Audio Visual Instruction.

Kohut, H. (1959). Introspection, empathy, and psychoanalysis: An examination of the relationship between mode of observation and theory. *Journal of the American Psychoanalytic Association, 7,* 459–483.

Kohut, H. (1971). *The analysis of the self: A systematic approach to the psychoanalytic treatment of narcissistic personality disorders.* New York: International Universities Press.

Kohut, H. (1984). *How does analysis cure?* Chicago: University of Chicago Press.

Kris, E. (1950). On preconscious mental processes. In E. Kris, The selected papers of Ernst Kris (pp. 217–236). New Haven, CT: Yale University Press, 1975.

Kris, E. (1951). Ego psychology and interpretation in psychoanalytic therapy. In E. Kris, *The selected papers of Ernst Kris* (pp. 237–251). New Haven, CT: Yale University Press, 1975.

Kris, E. (1956a). On some vicissitudes of insight in psychoanalysis. *International Journal of Psycho-Analysis, 37,* 445–455.

Kris, E. (1956b). The recovery of childhood memories in psychoanalysis. In E. Kris, *The selected papers of Ernst Kris.* (pp. 301–340). New Haven, CT: Yale University Press, 1975.

Langs, R. (1979). *The technique of psychoanalytic psychotherapy.* New York: Jason Aronson.

Langs, R. (1979). *The therapeutic environment.* New York: Jason Aronson.

Lichtenberg, J. (1983a). *Psychoanalysis and infant research.* Hillsdale, NJ: Analytic Press.

Lichtenberg, J. (1983b). The influence of values and value judgment on the psychoanalytic encounter. *Psychoanalytic Inquiry, 3,* 647–664.

Lichtenberg, J. (1989). Psychoanalysis and motivation. Hillsdale, NJ: Analytic Press.

Linsner, J. P. (1987). Therapeutically effective and ineffective insight: The immediate effects of therapist behavior on a patient's insight during short-term dynamic therapy (Doctoral dissertation, City University of New York). *Dissertation Abstracts International,* 1988, *48*(12b). (University Microfilms No. 88-01,731).

Lipton, S. (1967). Later developments in Freud's technique (1920–1939). In B. Wolman (Ed.), *Psychoanalytic techniques: A handbook for practicing psychoanalysts* (pp. 51–92). New York: Basic Books.

Loewald, H. (1960). On the therapeutic action of psychoanalysis. *International Journal of Psycho-Analysis, 41,* 17–33.

Loewald, H. (1979). The waning of the Oedipus complex. *Journal of the American Psychoanalytic Association, 27,* 751–775.

Loewenstein, R. M. (1954). Some remarks on defenses, autonomous ego and psychoanalytic technique. *International Journal of Psycho-Analysis, 35,* 188–193.

Lomas, P. (1982). *The limits of interpretation.* Northvale, NJ: Jason Aronson.

Luborsky, L. (1988). *Who will benefit from psychotherapy?* New York: Basic Books.

Mahl, G. F. (1956). Disturbances and silences in the patient's speech in psychotherapy. *Journal of Abnormal and Social Psychology, 53*, 1–15.

Modell, A. (1965). On having the right to a life: An aspect of the superego's development. *International Journal of Psycho-Analysis, 46*, 323–331.

Modell, A. (1971). The origin of certain forms of pre-Oedipal guilt and the implications for a psychoanalytic theory of affects. *International Journal of Psycho-Analysis, 52*, 337–346.

Norville, R. (1989). Plan compatibility of interpretations and brief psychotherapy outcome (Doctoral dissertation, Pacific Graduate School of Psychology). *Dissertation Abstracts International, 50*(12), 5888B. (University Microfilms No. 90-12,770)

O'Connor, L., Edelstein, S., Berry J., & Weiss, J. (Submitted for publication). The pattern of insight in brief psychotherapy: A series of pilot studies.

Persons, J. (1989). *Cognitive therapy in practice. A case formulation approach.* New York: Norton.

Rangell, L. (1969a). The intrapsychic process and its analysis: A recent line of thought and its current implications. *International Journal of Psycho-Analysis, 50*, 65–77.

Rangell, L. (1969b). Choice, conflict, and the decision-making function of the ego: A psychoanalytic contribution to decision theory. *International Journal of Psycho-Analysis, 50*, 599–602.

Rangell, L. (1981a). From insight to change. *Journal of the American Psychoanalytic Association, 29*, 119–141.

Rangell, L. (1981b). Psychoanalysis and dynamic psychotherapy: Similarities and differences twenty-five years later. *Psychoanalytic Quarterly, 50*, 665–693.

Ransohoff, P., Drucker, C., & Sampson, F. (1987, December). *Changes a patient makes during analysis: An empirical demonstration.* Paper presented at the annual meeting of the American Psychoanalytic Association. New York.

Rosenberg, S., Silberschatz, G., Curtis, J., Sampson, H., & Weiss, J. (1986). The plan diagnosis method: A new approach to establishing reliability for psychodynamic formulations. *American Journal of Psychiatry, 143*(11), 1454–1456.

Shilkret, C., Isaacs, M., Drucker, C., & Curtis, J. T. (1986). The acquisition of insight. In J. Weiss, H. Sampson, & the Mount Zion Psychotherapy Research Group (Eds.), *The psychoanalytic process: Theory, clinical observation & empirical research* (pp. 206–217). New York: Guilford Press.

Silberschatz, G., Sampson, H., & Weiss, J. Testing pathogenic beliefs versus seeking transference gratifications. In J. Weiss, H. Sampson, & the Mount Zion Psychotherapy Research Group (Eds.), *The psychoanalytic process: Theory, clinical observation & empirical research* (pp. 267–276). New York: Guilford Press.

Silberschatz, G., & Curtis, J. T. (1986). Clinical implications of research on brief dynamic psychotherapy: II. How the therapist helps or hinders therapeutic progress. *Psychoanalytic Psychology, 3*(1), 27–37.

Silberschatz, G., & Curtis, J.T. (in press). Measuring the therapist's impact on the patient's therapeutic progress. *Journal of Consulting and Clinical Psychology.*

Silberschatz, G., Fretter, P., & Curtis, J. (1986). How do interpretations influence the process of psychotherapy? *Journal of Consulting and Clinical Psychology, 54*(5), 646–652.

Stern, D. (1985). *The interpersonal world of the infant: A view from psychoanalysis and developmental psychology.* New York: Basic Books, 1985.

Stolorow, R. D., & Lachmann, F. M. (1984–1985). Transference: The future of an illusion. *Annual of Psychoanalysis, 12–13,* 19–37.

Strachey, J. (1934). The nature of the therapeutic action of psychoanalysis. *International Journal of Psycho-Analysis, 15,* 127–159.

Sullivan, H. S. (1940). Conceptions of modern psychiatry: The first William Alanson White Memorial Lectures. *Psychiatry, 3*(1), 1–117.

Thoma, H., & Kachele, H. (1992). *Psycho-analytic practice: Two clinical studies.* Berlin: Springer-Verlag.

Wallerstein, R. S. (1986). *Forty-two lives in treatment: A study of psychoanalysis and psychotherapy.* New York: Guilford Press.

Weinshel, E. M. (1970). The ego in health and normality. *Journal of the American Psychoanalytic Association, 18,* 682–735.

Weiss, J. (1971). The emergence of new themes: A contribution to the psychoanalytic theory of therapy. *International Journal of Psycho-Analysis, 52*(4), 459–467.

Weiss, J. (1952). Crying at the happy ending. *Psychoanalytic Review, 39*(4), 338.

Weiss, J. (1990). Unconscious mental functioning. *Scientific American, 262*(3), 103–109.

Weiss, J. (1992, June). *Our studies of the changes in the patient's level of insight in brief psychotherapy.* Paper presented at the annual meeting of the Society for Psychotherapy Research, Berkeley, CA.

Weiss, J. (in press). Empirical studies of the therapeutic process. *Journal of the American Psychoanalytic Association.*

Weiss, J., Sampson, H., & the Mount Zion Psychotherapy Research Group. (1986). *The psychoanalytic process: Theory, clinical observations and empirical research.* New York: Guilford Press.

Winnicott, D. W. (1965). *The maturational processes and the facilitating environment: Studies in the theory of emotional development.* New York: International Universities Press.

Winson, J. (1990). The meaning of dreams. *Scientific American, 262*(3), 86–96.

Zahn-Waxler, C., & Radke-Yarrow, M. (1982). The development of altruism: Alternative research strategies. In N. Eisenberg (Ed.), *The development of pro-social behavior* (pp. 109–137). San Diego: Academic Press.

Zetzel, E. R., & Meissner, W. W. (1973). *Basic concepts of psychoanalytic psychiatry*. New York: Basic Books.

Index

n indicates that entry will be found in a footnote